HCG Diet

Losing Weight
One Phase at a Time©

A Simplified Guide Book
With Motivational Charts

Carla Martell & Audrey Scott

Copyright Statement

Caricature Artwork by Victor Alexander Dorobantu
www.MyCaricature.com

Cover Design by Douglas A. Teeples
www.ArtisticPortraits.com *"Realistic Hand-Painted Oil Portraits from Photographs"*

Published by Cluster Storm Publishing. U.S.A. No part of this book may be used or reproduced in any manner whatsoever without the written permission of the authors.

ISBN 1-56998-003-9

Printed by
dmt PUBLISHING
900 North 400 West #12
North Salt Lake, UT 84054
www.dmtpublishing.com

Table of Contents

Disclaimers

This book is intended to inform, motivate and guide you in your personal journey through the HCG protocol as described by Dr. Simeons in *"Pounds and Inches"*.

We are not medical doctors and the information in this book is not intended to provide medical advice, diagnose illness or in any way attempt to practice medicine. This information is also not intended to replace personal medical care and advice from a licensed physician.

It is recommended that you check with your physician before beginning any weight loss program. If you have any additional concerns or questions regarding your own health, you should seek medical assistance for a licensed health care practitioner.

Dedications

I would like to express a huge thank you to my husband Lance for the many hours of research and editing that went into this book. Lance and my children have been my cheerleaders and my motivation for making this project successful. I love you all.

Carla Martell

Thank you Dean for believing in this project and for even trying the diet yourself so you could see that it can really be successful. I guess by losing 25 pounds in three weeks, I convinced you that it is not a farce. Thanks for the love and support you have given me and my sister, so we were able to make this book possible.

Audrey Scott

We would also like to acknowledge and commend Dr. A. T. W. Simeons for his research and discoveries in a weight loss protocol that quite simply works with lifelong success.

Foreward by Dr. Turner:

Have you wondered if you can *really* do the HcG Diet? This book and the companion HcG recipes book are valuable tools that can help you succeed. We have been prescribing HcG at the Jordan Health and Wellness Center for many years.

The HcG Diet is not the only successful weight loss program we use, but without a doubt, it is the most rapid method available for losing body fat. I, too, was skeptical when I first learned about HcG, but after studying Dr. Simeon's work and meeting people who successfully lost weight and kept it off for more than 20 years, well…results speak for themselves.

HcG is not without controversy. Any practitioner or healing modality that might interfere with the economics of the sick care model that is the standard healthcare status quo will find an academic and political bias against that person or therapy. HcG is one of those therapies. A better understanding of the biochemistry of HcG is certainly needed. However, waiting for that information in an era of bias when the therapy is experientially safe and effective does not make sense.

Over sixty-six degenerative diseases including diabetes and certain cancers are directly linked to obesity. Losing fat can not only save billions of dollars in health care costs to society, it can improve your quality of life and possibly save your life. Bariatric surgeons are touting the concept that gastric bypass surgery might cure diabetes. Why choose the blade when you can safely reduce body fat without surgery?

With fewer medication requirements, an HcG protocol will not put synthetic chemicals into your body and will help you maintain a healthier acid-base balance. Proper pH in your tissues is believed to reduce your risk of disease burden. With weight loss, you are more motivated to exercise and adopt other healthy lifestyle habits that go further to improve your quality of life. Working with a renowned body builder, we learned that if a person has more than 30 pounds to lose, the physical training necessary to build the muscle mass required to maintain your ideal weight is just impossible.

Losing fat is the first step to vitality and longevity. While most people following any diet program will not make all the changes needed to lose the fat, build muscle mass to the ideal fat-to-muscle ratio and make all the lifestyle adjustments needed to maintain a lifetime of ideal health, losing fat can alone do wonders for your overall health.

Carla and Audrey have written a wonderful guide to successfully follow the Simeon HcG diet protocol. The meals in the companion recipes book are also designed to stay within Dr. Simeon's original work. Others, without real thought, have created diets and recipes that stray from Dr. Simeon's research and may lead HcG patients away from their best successes. By following the advice in these books, you too, can lose fat, change your health and live with vitality. You *can* do the HcG Diet, and you will be amazed by the results.

Dr. Bryan Turner, DVM, MD

The Jordan Health and Wellness Center is the premier holistic and integrative medical center along Utah's Wasatch Front. The Professionals at Jordan Health are passionate about delivering wholistic and responsible treatments to their patients. Medical weight loss, attention to cardiovascular health, and reducing the risk factors for heart attacks, and strokes are important parts of the Center's approach to wholebody health. Natural hormone therapies and thyroid evaluation are of particular focus in Dr. Turner's work at the Center. www.jordanhealthandwellness.com
 blog:www.bryanturnermd.wordpress.com

Before starting the HCG Protocol

1. We ask anyone considering the HCG protocol to read all of Dr. Simeons' manuscript, *"Pounds and Inches: A New Approach to Obesity"*, which is printed at the end of this book. Familiarize yourself with Dr. Simeons' protocol so you can more fully understand the things we have written in this book. Dr. Simeons gives exact information about the research he conducted in regards to curing obesity. In our opinion, he succeeded in finding a cure! He has given us the guidelines necessary to free you of the challenges and complications of excess weight. This weight loss can last a lifetime by getting rid of stored fat and resetting your metabolism.

2. You should always check with your physician before beginning any weight loss program. At this time you should also discuss any additional medications you are taking.

3. To proceed forward with the HCG protocol you will need to acquire HCG whether in drops, spray, injections, etc. If you are taking HCG by injections you will need to get a prescription from a doctor.

4. You will need to acquire a quality digital bathroom scale that measures pounds to the tenth and a quality food scale that measures in grams.

5. Decide when you want to start Phase 2. Start the protocol at a time when Phase 2 and/or 3 will not run interference with a trip or a holiday that involves a lot of eating (you know which ones they are!)

6. If you are a menstruating, refer to page 22 regarding when to avoid starting Phase 2 of the protocol.

7. If you are taking HCG by injections or HCG powder, mix your solution the day before you plan on starting Phase 2 and store it in the refrigerator. Do not mix the solution before this time. If you are taking HCG by pre-mixed drops or spray, no preliminary mixing is necessary. (Full instructions are found in Chapter 2.)

8. Take your body measurements and record them on the Measurement Tracking Log on page 96. Take "before" pictures from front, side and back profile. If you are brave enough, paste them into this book on page 97. We recommend you do this because the "after" pictures are going to be incredible. The two pictures side by side will be great for your motivation.

9. Stock your refrigerator with natural meats, fruits and veggies as listed in Chapter 3 under Phase 2. (Refer to shopping list, page 7)

10. Good luck in your adventure through this protocol. Go forward and enjoy the new you!

Shopping List

Sweetener options

Stevia	Found at your local grocery or health food store
Stevia flavored drops	Found at health food store or online
Truvia	Found at your local grocery or health food store

Drinks Options

Coffee (optional)   Mineral water
Fresh lemon   Perrier sparkling water
Fresh lime   Tea (optional)
Herbal Teas

Meat, Chicken, or Seafood Options

Brisket   Lobster   Veal
Chicken breast (skinless/boneless)   Roast beef
Crab   Shrimp
Ground beef   Steak
Ground chicken   White fish

Vegetable Options

Asparagus   Fennel
Beet Greens   Lettuce (of any kind)
Cabbage   Onions (yellow or red)
Celery   Radishes
Chard   Spinach
Cucumbers   Tomatoes
Fennel   Chicory

Fruit Options

Apple   Oranges
Grapefruit   Strawberries

Melba Toast or Breadsticks

Melba toast- (original, or Garlic)
Grissini Breadsticks (original, or Garlic)

Spice & Seasoning Options

Allspice	Garlic powder
Apple cider vinegar	Green onions
Bay leaves	Italian seasoning
Bragg's liquid aminos	Jalapeño
Cayenne pepper	Marjoram
Celery salt	McCormick Italian Seasoning
Chili powder	Nutmeg
Chinese Five Spice Powder	Onion flakes
Chipotle seasoning	Onion powder
Cilantro	Oregano
Cinnamon	Paprika
Cumin	Parsley
Curry powder	Pepper
Dill weed	Sage
Dried red pepper	Savory
Dry mustard	Sea salt
Fresh ginger	Thyme
Fresh rosemary	Wrights liquid smoke
Garlic	

Miscellaneous Options

Miracle Noodles	Found at www.miraclenoodles.com
Konjac flour	Found at www.konjacfoods.com
Tomato sauce	
Tomato paste	
Milk	

Helpful Kitchen Tools

Blender	Grill	Food Processer
George Forman Grill	Juicer	

Items can be absorbed into the skin and can affect the diet while on HCG. Below is a list of products that are proven safe and we have listed where you can find them.

Product Category   Where to Find Items

Cosmetics

Mineral makeup	Department stores, Costco, Salons
Oil-free foundation	Drug stores, Department stores

Face Cleaners

Neutrogena Oil Free Cleanser	Drug stores, Retail stores
Witch Hazel	Drug stores, Retail stores
Clean & Clear	Drug stores, Retail stores
Clearasil oil free gel cleanser	Drug stores, Retail stores

Toothpaste

Tom's of Maine Toothpaste	Health food store, Drug stores
Spry Toothpaste	Health food store, Internet

Deodorant

Crystal Deodorant	Health food store, Retail stores

Shampoos/Conditioners

Magick Botanicals oil free	Internet
Desert Essence Organics	Internet
Jason oil free	Internet
Natures Gate Aloe Vera	Internet, Health food stores
Herbal oil free	Internet

Body Soaps

Zum Bar	Health food stores, Internet
Organic oil free soaps	Health food stores, Internet
Dial	Drug stores, Retail stores
Zest	Drug stores, Retail stores
Ivory	Drug stores, Retail stores

Dr. Simeons' Story

Dr. Simeons was a world renowned physician born in England in the early part of the last century. He was trained in Europe and spent 18 years in India helping to study and combat tropical diseases.

After World War II, Dr. Simeons became interested in the problem of obesity. At that time, in post war Europe and America, obesity was a rare phenomenon. Because of its rarity, and partly because of the fact that it was increasingly becoming a problem in Western society, Dr. Simeons was attracted to the problem.

He began research into the problem of obesity and made some astounding discoveries. A couple of observations he made in India while studying tropical diseases led him to create some key theories and eventually develop a protocol for managing obesity in humans.

In India, one of the poorest countries in the world, Dr. Simeons observed that the babies born to women would be healthy and full size even though the mother might be 'surviving' on less food than was thought sufficient to support a fetus. Even though the mother might consume only 500 calories, the baby would be born healthy and full weight. How could this be? How could the mother's body produce a full size healthy baby on such a sparse diet?

Dr. Simeons discovered the role of HCG in human fetal development. When a woman is pregnant her body begins to produce a hormone called human chorionic gonadotrophin (HCG). This hormone directs the metabolism of the mother to begin burning stored fat to feed that energy to the fetus. With this hormone driven energy charge, the mother's body sacrifices fat in order to feed the developing baby.

Consequently, a woman living on rations considered to be starvation level in the West today, could metabolically support a fetus to full term and produce a healthy full size infant. The woman would suffer significant fat loss but the baby would survive.

His second observation was in regards to so called 'fat-boys'. These were underdeveloped male children with female bodily characteristics such as wide hips, knock knees, etc. It was found that after treatment with HCG, the patient would begin to develop normally and proper muscle tone and male characteristics would appear.

After making these observations and theorizing about the role of HCG in human metabolism, Dr. Simeons set about developing a protocol to use HCG to help people combat obesity. His theory was that if HCG could be used to 'trick' the body into burning up excess stored fat, then obesity could be solved. After several years of painstaking research, Dr. Simeons developed just such a protocol.

When Dr. Simeons published his findings to the medical world in 1954 he was rejected and condemned. In response, he opened his own clinic to treat overweight rich and powerful people in Europe and effectively took his knowledge underground.

About HCG

In scientific terms, HCG (Human Chorionic Gonadotrophin) is a glycoprotein and is composed of an alpha subunit and a beta subunit. HCG is closely related to two other gonadotropins; luteinizing hormone (LH) and follicle stimulating hormone (FSH). It is also related to thyroid stimulating hormone (TSH). All three of which are glycoprotein hormones.

In simpler terms, HCG is a natural hormone that is found in the human body. HCG is produced in a specific part of the placenta during a woman's pregnancy to help the unborn baby grow properly, to keep the ovary intact, and is involved in the production of progesterone which is important during pregnancy. Researchers also speculate that HCG boosts a woman's immune system during pregnancy.

HCG is used to treat several different medical problems in men and women such as infertility, hormone imbalances and as treatment for underdeveloped boys. This was actually what British physician, Dr. Simeons MD, was researching in the 1950's when he first noticed that the hormone was allowing the patients treated with HCG to lose fat but keep their muscle.

Fat Types

There are three types of fat in the human body. The first kind of fat is structural fat which provides protection for the body's major organs and joints and is not burned for metabolism. The second kind of fat is normal fat reserves which are spread all over the body. These first two types of fat are needed for good health.

The third kind of fat found in the body is called abnormal stored fat. This fat is kept in storage under the skin and around the organs as a "spare fuel supply." In an overweight person, it tends to collect in places like the hips, buttocks, upper arms, abdomen, knees, ankles and neck.

How HCG helps weight loss

Dr. Simeons believed that HCG keeps the structural fat and muscle intact while breaking down the abnormal body fat. The HCG hormone stimulates the glands of the body to use the excess abnormal fat. As the HCG metabolizes abnormal body fat, about 2,000 calories each day are released into the bloodstream. This allows a person to eat a low calorie diet, consisting of 500 calories, without experiencing fatigue, weakness or hunger. If you have ever had trouble losing weight from your hips or stomach with exercise and diet, it may be because it is abnormal fat and your body never wanted to use it for energy. This simply means it just stays on your body. When you take HCG with a low calorie diet, you use the fat that is hard to lose for fuel. Your problem areas, such as your hips and stomach become thinner first and quickly. Dr. Simeons believed the cause of obesity was an abnormally functioning hypothalamus. He believed the use of HCG along with a very low calorie diet also helped to re-set the hypothalamus to normal, thereby normalizing metabolism, appetite, and the storage of fat. Most importantly, by following this protocol, the weight and inches you lose will stay off when you're finished as long as a healthy diet is followed.

Chapter 1

HCG Diet at a Glance

We have put together a brief summary of the HCG Diet for quick reference. Full details about each Phase are outlined in Chapter 3.

To help make this diet easier to understand, we took each step from Dr. Simeons' HCG Protocol, numbered them and called it a "Phase". You should follow each Phase in order.

"The pessimist sees the difficulty in every opportunity; and the optimist sees the opportunity in every difficulty."

Winston Churchill

Phase 1 at a Glance:

Before you diet, it is suggested doing some kind of colon cleanse and/or detoxification. There are many different colon, metals and Candida cleansing products available. Check with your local nutritionist or health food store for suggested recommendations for these cleanses.

Phase 2 at a Glance:

- **(Day 1 & 2)** Weigh yourself in the morning. Take your HCG and gorge.

Start taking the HCG drops (10 – 15 drops, 3x a day) (or injections that are prescribed by a doctor or any other approved form of HCG). When using HCG drops, start with 10 drops - 3 times a day. If you feel too hungry or weak, you can increase up to 15 drops each time – giving you 45 drops a day. You may also take 23 drops in the morning and 22 drops at night, taking the drops only twice a day. If you take more than 60 drops a day it does not make the HCG work faster. In fact, you can actually slow down your weight loss progress if you take too many drops.

The drops go under your tongue. Try to hold the drops under the tongue 1 – 3 minutes before swallowing. Do not eat or drink or brush your teeth within 15 minutes before or after taking the drops.

During the first 2 days of HCG you need to gorge on fatty foods. Eat as much as you can throughout the day. The more you eat these 2 days and the higher the fat content, the better.

- **(Day 3-23 or up to 40 days)** Take your HCG.

Continue to weigh yourself every morning (recording your weight) and take the HCG drops 2 or 3x a day. (Do not take HCG during a menstrual cycle.)

Drink at least 1/2 gallon or (8) 9oz water bottles throughout the day. Water is critical to help flush the fat from your body.

Stay on the 500 calorie diet for the remainder of phase 2.

Eat only from the food lists starting on page 26. Do not skip meals. Your total intake will be about 500 calories consisting of protein, vegetables and fruit. (Remember that the HCG drops will release an additional 1500 calories into your system.

Do not do any strenuous exercising during phase 2.

- **(Last 3 days of Phase 2)** Stop the HCG but continue the 500 Calorie Diet.

Phase 3 at a Glance:

Part One: Continue to weigh yourself each morning. Begin eating a full calorie diet (1500 calories a day) eating any food at this point, except all starches and sugars*. If the scale shows more than 2 pounds over the weight you were on the last day of Phase 2, do a "steak day" (as described on page 32). It is important to continue Part One of Phase 3 for three weeks. Most people don't realize how vital this part is in resetting the hypothalamus. You will be establishing a new set point for your weight. By doing this, your body will not put all the weight back on you just lost, when you return to normal eating.

* For a complete list of starches and sugars refer to pages 34 and 35.

Part Two: Slowly start adding starches and sugar, in small quantities, to your diet. The key to this is slowly! Continue weighing yourself every morning to control weight gain. If your weight goes up 2 pounds, a steak day will bring the weight down to the desired weight.

Phase 4 at a Glance:

Most importantly during the Maintenance Phase, you need to relax and eat mindfully. Learn to be aware of food and what causes you to turn to food for the wrong reasons. What you eat and how you eat can help or harm you.

Learn to manage stress. Start a routine of relaxation/fitness techniques such as Yoga, Meditation, Tai Chi, Visualization etc.   Remember, stress generates cortisol which in turn makes your body store fat. Learn to let go of stress as this will not only help you to be happier but also to stay thinner.

Now is the beginning of a new way of life! Use the motivation of your new body to create and continue good habits of healthy eating and <u>regular</u> exercise. Doing so will maintain your weight for life. Enjoy yourself as a healthier, happier you.

"Life is not going to hand you
what you want;
you're going to have to create it."

Richard E. Goldman

Chapter 2

Preparing the HCG

"All the wonders you seek are within yourself."

Sir Thomas Brown

Preparing the HCG

There are several ways you can take HCG. Our personal favorite method is the pre-mixed Homeopathic HCG drops. They eliminate the need to get a prescription and mix the solution yourself. There is no difference between injected and HCG drops. Once HCG is in your body, it works exactly the same no matter how it gets there. The body does not know the difference between injected HCG and liquid HCG drops, it only acknowledges HCG and doesn't know where it came from. The following are three of the most common forms of HCG but new preparations are being developed all the time.

Injections: If you are taking HCG by injections, have your pharmacist mix it for you no sooner than 1 or 2 days before starting Phase 2.

HCG Powder: If you are using Sublingual HCG Powder, that is not pre-mixed, we have the following instructions we obtained from a doctor. "Use a brown glass bottle with a dropper top for mixing and storing the HCG solution. Rinse out the new bottle with filtered water. Then use about 1 ml (which is equal to 1 cc) of vodka to rinse your mixing bottle and pour the vodka down the sink. Add about 0.5 ml of vodka into the HCG ampoule to dissolve the powder. Pour the HCG powder mixed with the vodka into the mixing bottle and add 2.5 ml of vodka. After that, add enough distilled water to have a total of 20 ml of liquid. You can add 2-3 ml of B-12 liquid before adding the distilled water but if you do this, be sure the B-12 liquid does not contain any sugar or fructose syrup. (It is not necessary to add B-12.) If you buy 5000 i.u. vials, you will end up with a mixture containing 250 i.u. per ml." After mixing HCG, <u>do not shake.</u> Gently swirl the vial to mix powder and liquid.

Pre-mixed Homeopathic HCG Drops: With the Pre-mixed drops, no preparation is necessary. Just open the bottle and put drops under your tongue. Take a total of 36 – 45 drops each day, 2 or three times a day. The HCG drops method usually results in about half (50%) of the dose being absorbed into the bloodstream, so your doses are taken more than once a day. Also getting that 50% depends on how long you hold the HCG mix under your tongue. Try to hold it under your tongue at least 2 - 5 minutes each time before swallowing.

Chapter 3

The 4 Phases of the HCG Protocol

The following chapter outlines in detail the 4 Phases involved with following the HCG diet protocol as outlined in Dr. Simeons' manuscript "Pounds & Inches". (Refer to his manuscript at the end of this book.)

There are some things written in regards to the HCG Diet that are conflicting in information and instruction. Our philosophy is that if you are going to do Dr. Simeons' protocol, you need to do the program as *he* wrote it. We have thoroughly studied his manuscript and research results. With confidence in accuracy, we have written simple instructions that are easy to follow.

"We cannot become what we need to be by remaining what we are."

Max De Pree

Phase 1 - Preparation

Dr. Simeons' original HCG Protocol did not require a body detoxification period. But it has been recommended by several sources in recent years that a colon cleanse or a Candida cleanse is helpful to do for a couple of weeks before starting the HCG. It is widely believed that with the many toxins and chemicals we now come in contact with every day, regular body cleanses are a good idea whether or not you do the HCG diet.

We have labeled this cleansing phase as Phase 1. Of course, any diversion from Dr. Simeons' HCG Protocol is always optional and not required to be successful. Yet some people find cleanses to be helpful in "jump starting" Phase 2.

Phase 2 - HCG

1. Phase 2 consists of HCG intake and a very low calorie diet (500 calories a day). Don't panic when you read "500 calories". You need to remember that even though you are eating only 500 calories a day, you are actually getting around 2000 calories a day. This is because the HCG causes your reserved fat cells to release about 1500 calories into your system each day you are taking it. With the HCG you are able to eat a small amount but not feel as if you are starving. This is also why you can lose weight and inches so quickly and effectively without looking gaunt or drawn.

2. Phase 2 is done anywhere from 26 to 48 days. But the key thing to understand is that HCG is not taken every day during Phase 2. Let me explain why. Phase 2 is a minimum of 23 HCG intake days. Days 23 – 26 you will still eat the 500 calorie diet but not take HCG. The 48 maximum days of Phase 2, referred to above, consists of 40 days of taking HCG, 5 extra days for skipping HCG (once a week) and the 3 final days of continuing the 500 calorie diet with no HCG.

    Let us explain further. If you have 20 pounds to lose or less, you will probably want to do the 26 day program. The first 23 days you will take

HCG (every day) while doing the 500 calorie diet with very specific foods. (The diet requirements for Phase 2 are outlined on pg 25.) The last 3 days, of the 26 day round, are done with the 500 calorie diet but no HCG. This is done so that all the HCG is sure to be out of your system before you begin eating full calories.

Take note, even if you need to lose only 5 - 10 pounds you will still do the 26 days of Phase 2. Dr. Simeons never gave a treatment lasting less than 26 days. He wrote that even in the mildest cases of necessary weight loss, your body needs a minimum of 23 days of HCG to "set" the glands. If not, the weight will easily be regained.

If you need to lose more than 20 pounds, you will want to do Phase 2 somewhere between 26 - 48 days. If you are doing a 48 day round, you will take HCG only 40 of the days. You do this by taking HCG for 6 straight days, then skipping the 7th day. Repeat this until you've taken your HCG a total of 40 days.

Dr. Simeons found that no more than 40 doses of HCG should be taken in one round. Immunity to the HCG may begin to build up if it's taken longer. This will cause your weight loss to slow down or stop.

The 500 calorie diet is done every day of this phase – even on the days you don't take HCG, with the exception of the last 3 days of Phase 2. Those 3 days you will not take HCG but the 500 calorie diet continues. Again the final 3 days of dieting with no HCG is necessary to get all the HCG out of your system. If you start to eat normally on those last 3 days, with even a trace of HCG in your body, you will put on weight quickly at the end of the phase.

3. Dr. Simeons also found that no more than 34 pounds should be lost in one round of Phase 2. The exception to this rule is if the person is extremely obese, he/she may be allowed to lose an additional 5 – 6 pounds as long as the weight is lost before the 40 doses of HCG are taken. **You should stop at 34 pounds or 40 doses, whichever comes first.** If you need to lose more weight after completing Phase 2, a second round of Phase 2 can be done after waiting at least 6 weeks. It takes 6 weeks after using HCG before the immunity to it is diminished and HCG becomes fully effective again.

4. During the 6 week waiting time, you should do 6 weeks of Phase 3. Then you may do Phase 2 again for a 26 – 48 day round. When a third, fourth, or even fifth round is necessary, the waiting interval between each round should be made progressively longer.

5. Dr. Simeons recommended that women do not take the HCG during their menstrual cycle. If you find yourself feeling weak or hungry without taking the HCG during menstruation, try avoiding it only on the heaviest days of your cycle.

6. For the first couple of days of starting Phase 2, some people feel a little tired or weak while adjusting to the HCG and the 500 calorie diet, but after a week at the most, you should not feel badly. If you start to feel extremely weak after you have been doing Phase 2 awhile, the problem may be the potency of the HCG. The cause could also be immunity issues or you have achieved your ideal weight.

7. The rate of weight loss varies from person to person, but this is due to differences in body chemistry, NOT the method of taking your HCG. An individual person will very likely lose the same amount and at the same rate regardless of method, assuming they are doing it correctly.

Days 1 & 2 of Phase 2 (Gorge days)

- **First thing in the morning weigh yourself**

It is important to weigh yourself approximately the same time each morning, without clothes. Use a digital scale that measures to the tenth of a pound. Record your weight in your daily journal pages. (Starting on page 48.)

- **Taking HCG**

Start your HCG on day 1 even though you are not on the low calorie diet for the first two days of Phase 2

If you are taking HCG by injections, get instructions from your physician or pharmacist on how to administer the shots.

1. For HCG injections, the recommended dosage is 125 i.u. of HCG per day, according to Dr. Simeons. You only increase the daily dosage to

200 i.u. if you are not losing weight or are extremely hungry. If taken properly, 125 i.u. per dose is usually sufficient.

2. With HCG drops, place 12 – 15 drops under your tongue and hold there for at least 2 – 3 minutes but up to 5 minutes. Take HCG in this manner 3 times a day.

   Instead of taking HCG three times a day, you can take it 2 times a day, 18 – 23 drops in the morning and 18 – 22 drops in the evening.

   Don't eat or drink water or brush your teeth within 15 minutes before or after taking the drops.

- **Eat – a lot!**

The first two days we call "gorge" days. And you need to do exactly that – gorge, indulge, and knock yourself out! The more fattening foods you eat the better results you are going to have. Those who do not load their bodies to the fullest during the two gorge days tend to experience difficult hunger pains during some of Phase 2. Do <u>not</u> try to limit your food during these days as this step is important to re-establish the structural fat that's been reduced or lost by years of yo-yo dieting. Also the 2 days of gorging is what allows your body's fat reserve to open up & start releasing extra calories throughout Phase 2.

You will and <u>should</u> gain weight on the 2 gorge days but don't worry. You will lose it all within the first week; probably even the first day or two! Eat foods that you crave that are especially high in fat such as cheesecake, cookies, ice cream, pastries, chocolate, creamy soups, fried meats, eggs, and bacon to name a few. You can drink whatever you want on the gorge days, including soda.

It may seem hard to load yourself with really fatty, unhealthy items (especially if you're on your second or third round of the protocol), so here is a list of healthy items you can gorge on that are high in fat.

- ❖ Avocados
- ❖ Olives
- ❖ Breads
- ❖ Nuts - Especially Walnuts, Macadamia Nuts, Pecans, Cashews
- ❖ Seeds - Sesame, Sunflower, Pumpkin
- ❖ Salad dressing

Days 3 – 45

- **As in Day 1-2, weigh yourself first thing in the morning.**

Again, record your weight on your daily journal page. Always use a digital scale when weighing yourself.

- **Take your HCG.**

HCG is taken every morning with the following exceptions: If you are doing Phase 2 longer than 23 days, Dr. Simeons recommends you take HCG 6 days and skip 1 day. Skipping a day every 6 days will enable you to go longer on the HCG without building up immunity to it.

- **Start your 500 calorie diet as outlined on pages 26 - 28.**

- **The last 72 hours of Phase 2 do <u>NOT</u> take HCG but stay on the 500 Calorie diet.**

Continuing the 500 calorie eating for 72 more hours will assure that all the HCG is out of your system before you start eating more calories. For example, if you take your last HCG drops on Sunday morning at 9 am, you will begin the maintenance phase on Wednesday morning at 9 am.

500 Calorie Diet Menu

This is the 500 calorie a day plan that was outlined by Dr. Simeons in his manuscript *'Pounds and Inches'*. (Found at the end of this book.) It is the very low calorie diet required while taking HCG which starts on the third day of Phase 2. It has very specific foods and amounts.

Beverages

The drinks listed below are allowed all day in any amount with no sugar. Only one tablespoonful of milk is allowed in 24 hours. Any flavor stevia or Truvia may be used for a sweetener.

You should <u>drink ½ your weight in ounces, of water each day</u>. For example: If you weigh 140 lbs., drink 70 oz. Drinking more water does not make you retain water. The body is more likely to retain water when it has less that it needs. Don't drink any beverage that has artificial sweeteners even if they have zero calories. Only drink liquids from the following list.

Tea	**Coffee**	**Herbal tea**
Plain water	**Mineral water**	**Green tea**

Breakfast

Drink only from the list of beverages above. You can drink as much as you like.

Lunch

Eat only 100 grams of your choice of meat from the following list. All visible fat must be removed before cooking. Meat should be weighed before cooking. Broil, bake, grill or boil your meat. Cooking spray may be used, but no added fat. Salmon, eel, tuna, herring, lunch meats, dried or pickled fish are not allowed.

Beef	**Fresh white fish**	**Crab**	**Veal**
Chicken breast	**Lobster**	**Shrimp**	

Choose only one type of vegetable from the following list, eating only about a handful size portion. Do not mix the vegetables during one meal.

Green salad	**Celery**	**Radishes**
Spinach	**Onions**	**Chard**
Asparagus	**Tomatoes**	**Chicory**
Cucumbers	**Cabbage**	**Beet-greens**
Fennel		

You can have one Melba toast portion and one of your fruits during lunch or in between lunch and dinner.

1 breadstick (grissini)
1 Melba toast

Apple	**Half grapefruit**
Handful of strawberries	**Orange**

1 lemon or 1 lime per day

Dinner

Follow the same instructions as the lunch menu. Do not eat the same meat or the same fruit twice in one day.

Seasonings

The following seasonings are allowed. Make sure the seasonings do not contain MSG or sugar. Do not use any oil, butter or dressing. Organic seasonings should be the first choice when possible.

Apple cider vinegar	Garlic powder
Bay leaves	Green onions
Bragg's liquid aminos	Italian seasoning
Cayenne pepper	Jalapeño
Celery salt	Marjoram
Chili powder	McCormick Italian Seasoning
Chipotle seasoning	Nutmeg
Cilantro	Onion flakes
Cinnamon	Onion powder
Cumin	Oregano
Curry powder	Paprika
Dill weed	Parsley
Dried red pepper	Pepper
Dry mustard	Sage
Fresh ginger	Savory
Fresh rosemary	Sea salt
Garlic	Thyme

You do not need to eat everything listed each day. You may skip a fruit, breadstick, vegetable, etc. But do not skip proteins or water. Water is very important in flushing out the body.

The fruit or the breadstick may be eaten between meals instead of with lunch or dinner, but not more than four items listed for lunch and dinner may be eaten at one meal. People who struggle with blood sugar problems find it helpful to eat one of the fruits in the morning and the other one mid-day. If you eat the fruit or Melba toast at a different time, again do not eat more than 2 a day.   Note that two small apples would still be higher calories than one large apple. No matter what the size of apple, eat just one.

Regulating personal items you use during Phase 2

Dr. Simeons wrote, "Most women find it hard to believe that fats, oils, creams, and ointments applied to the skin are absorbed and interfere with weight reduction by HCG just as if they had been eaten. This sensitivity to even such very minor increases in nutritional intake is a peculiar feature of the HCG method". Because of this increased sensitivity, Dr. Simeons recommends using only oil free lotion, soap, facial cleanser, and make-up that is made with only natural ingredients containing no lanolin or synthetic chemicals.

In reference to cosmetics, Dr. Simeons recommends that "no cosmetics other than lipstick, eyebrow pencil and powder may be used". Mascara is acceptable now since it is not manufactured with petroleum oil as it was 50 years ago. There are also many companies that manufacture oil-free mineral eye makeup and foundation that are also acceptable for Phase 2; i.e. Bare Essentials, Raw Minerals, etc. Refer to page 9 for a list of acceptable personal items and where they can be found.

Tips for losing your maximum weight and getting off a weight plateau

If you find your weight loss slowing down or staying on a plateau during Phase 2, don't give up. If your weight loss begins to slow down after you've been consistently losing weight, evaluate your diet to make sure you are not making some of these common mistakes.

- ✓ Do not drink diet drinks even though they have 0 calories - diet drinks of any type will hinder your weight loss.

- ✓ Weigh your protein <u>before</u> cooking it. Your 100 grams serving size can be quite a bit different if you weigh it after cooking it.

- ✓ Do not eat the same protein for lunch and dinner.

- ✓ Do not eat too much beef - many people increase their weight loss rate by eating more chicken and fish rather than beef every day.

✓ Do not mix vegetables at a meal.

✓ Make sure seasonings don't contain sugar or MSG

✓ Do not chew gum or suck on mints.

✓ Drink plenty of water - you should drink at least 2 - 4 quarts of liquid per day.

You may still lose weight if you are not adhering to each rule, but you will lose more consistently if you follow Dr. Simeons' protocol exactly.

Your weight may also plateau for a few days. Don't dismay. If you are doing everything right and have avoided the pitfalls listed above, you can try some of the following tips to accelerate weight loss:

✓ Cut down on the amount of beef you eat

✓ Be sure there are no additives in your chicken, fish or beef

✓ Don't eat the same fruit for both of your daily fruit intakes

✓ Eat a smaller apple as one of your fruits

✓ Try cutting out tomatoes, oranges or shrimp. These particular foods can occasionally slow weight loss on some individuals who may be sensitive to it. You can experiment to see if this is a problem by cutting out one food item at a time for several days. If weight loss is the same, consider that food alright to eat. But when you stop eating a particular food and notice significant weight loss, stop eating the food that caused your sensitivity.

✓ Cut out one or both of the breadsticks/melba toasts

✓ Increase your water intake

✓ You can add 1 or 2 glasses of green tea or take green tea capsules

✓ Use Smooth Move tea if you have trouble with constipation

If you still show no weight loss after 4 days and are doing everything right, you may have an "apple day" to get off the plateau and start losing again.

Apple Day:

An apple day consists of eating only 6 organic apples for that day. Drink a small amount of water, just enough to quench your thirst when needed. There should be a drop in weight the next morning but if there isn't don't worry. You need to remember that at times there may be no change in results on the scale but your body is still losing inches.

One of the key benefits of losing weight with Dr. Simeons' Protocol is that your body will not only lose weight but will lose it from the correct places. As the 'excess' fat is lost and the beneficial 'structural' fat is retained, those places on your body where unwanted fat has accumulated will be 'reshaped.' You will find that the fat deposits on your hips, thighs, stomach, arms, buttocks, and legs will disappear as you progress through the protocol. The accumulation of unwanted fat will diminish as the invaluable 'structural' fat that your body needs to stay healthy will be rebuilt.

Remember that the important structural fat is in place to cushion and protect your organs, bones and joints. Be assured that even if you do not lose as much weight each day as you hope, you will still see your body change in positive ways as it is re-sculpted into its natural beautiful form.

Phase 3 – Stabilization

Congratulations are in order when you complete Phase 2 and reach Phase 3. This is an important phase of the diet and is part of Dr. Simeons' original protocol. Successfully following the instructions in this phase will result in resetting your metabolism to a normal state.

Phase 3 will cause your body to reset its weight to a 'normal' set point. It will also reset the hypothalamus clearing off all the past years of yo-yo dieting and poor eating habits. This will keep your metabolism regulated at a normal level. This normal hypothalamus level allows your body to burn off calories as they are taken in so you don't gain weight as easily.

Before you begin Phase 3, make sure you have recorded what your weight was the last day your HCG was taken. This will be your *"ending Phase 2 weight"*.

Part One

Days 1 – 21

- **Stop taking the HCG**

During this phase you will stop the HCG for at least 6 weeks total.

- **Continue to weigh yourself first thing in the morning.**

Keep a daily log of your weight and notes of what you eat and your exercise activity during Phase 3. A Phase 3 recording sheet is found on page 95.

Weighing yourself daily is very important. Because the hypothalamus is now corrected from its abnormal condition, when you gain weight the body will not store the excess in the abnormal fat reserves as it did before. Weight gain will now be distributed evenly throughout the body. This means that looking in the mirror, or by feeling how your clothes fit, will be misleading. You can actually gain ten pounds and never notice it. This is why daily weighing is important.

If the scale shows more than a 2 pound gain over your *ending Phase 2 weight*, you will do a "steak day" that same day. (See page 32) According to Dr. Simeons, this step is very important. If you do not follow Phase 3 exactly, your body will try to recover the weight that you just lost in Phase 2. This is the 'yo-yo' effect so often experienced with dieting.

Steak Day

The same day the scale goes beyond two pounds from your *ending Phase 2 weight*, you must entirely skip all food until 6:00 p.m. During this time you should drink as much water, up to one gallon, as you can. You must drink a minimum of half a gallon of purified water.

In addition to the water, drink as much of the various teas that are recommended. You may use Stevia or Truvia in the teas. In the evening eat the biggest steak you can.

The steak can be grilled or cooked in a skillet and seasoned with pepper and herbs, but no salt. With the steak, you may have either a large raw tomato or large raw apple.

The better you are at keeping your weight fluctuation in a very small range, the better and quicker your body will settle into its new weight set point.

On the flip side of gaining more than 2 pounds, Dr. Simeons also discovered that it is equally undesirable for you to lose more than two pounds below your *ending Phase 2 weight.* This is because any loss of weight after the last HCG dose is usually a loss of muscle, or structural fat.

Dr. Simeons observed that "some patients become overly enthusiastic after the success they achieved during Phase 2. These patients do not believe they can eat normal amounts of food each day without regaining weight. They disregard the advice to eat anything they please (with the short list of exceptions) and want to play it safe. They try, more or less, to continue the low calorie diet from Phase 2 with minor variations." When they do this, they find that their weight actually goes up.

Dr. Simeons explained the reason for this. He wrote, "During Phase 2 the patient is just above the verge of protein deficiency, but because of the HCG protein is being fed back into a system from the breakdown and release of the secure problem area fatty tissue."

He goes on to write, "Once the treatment is over, there is no more HCG in the body and this process no longer takes place. Unless an adequate amount of protein is eaten as soon as Phase 2 is over, protein deficiency is bound to develop. This inevitably causes a marked retention of water, increased weight, which many times results in swelling of the ankles, huge hunger, tiredness, and irritability."

- **Begin eating a full calorie diet (1500 calories a day) eating any food at this point, except all starches and sugars.**

When you start the 3 week maintenance/stabilization process, you will increase your calories to at least 1500.

Don't try to continue the 500 calorie diet after the HCG is out of your system, because you will become weak and tired, and your body will begin to go into 'starvation shutdown' mode where it doesn't burn calories. This will ruin your Phase 2 progress, and you'll need to start all over.

Remember that the HCG was releasing an additional 1500+ calories into your system the same time you ate 500 calories during Phase 2. Make sure you are eating enough. Some people think they need to keep eating like they're on a diet. Don't do this. It is crucial to eat plenty of protein. Use healthy fats and dairy products to up your calorie intake if necessary. Drink plenty of water.

Don't worry, your weight will go up and down a bit the first week or two; this is normal. You will do a steak day when you need to. (Refer to page 32) Your weight will eventually stabilize. This is your body setting its new set point. With that said, you still need to be aware of your appetite and not eat too much. Many people, out of habit, put large amounts of food on their plate.

During this time you will notice you get full very quickly. Take note of the feeling of fullness and loss of appetite and stop eating when you are full. Eat a full breakfast, lunch, and dinner, and have three snacks throughout the day, ideally consisting of an apple or a grapefruit.

- **No starch and sugar during Part One – The first 3 weeks.**

READ LABELS to see if sugar is added into a product before you buy it. Nearly all processed foods contain high fructose corn syrup or some other kind of sugar. Nearly every product in a can or box contains sugar in one of its many forms. Most restaurants and fast food places add sugar to nearly every product, so be wary of eating out too often.

Avoiding starch means to stay away from the following food items:

Cornstarch	Tortillas & taco	All winter squashes
White flour	shells	Lentils
Wheat flour	Oatmeal & all	Pretzels
All flour	cereals	Corn chips
Grains	Rice	All potato chips
Pasta	Polenta	Popcorn
Pancakes	Peas	Rice cake
Muffins	Corn	Nuts
All breads or bread	Beets	Processed meat
products	Yams	Processed cheese
Breading on protein	Potatoes	
Crackers	Beans	

Avoid all sugar.

Cookies	Soft drinks	Pudding
Cake	Corn syrup	Canned fruit in syrup
Pie	Kool-Aid	Ice cream
Candy	All sodas	Boxed breakfast cereals
Cupcakes	Energy drinks	Breakfast bars
Donuts	Fruit juice	Granola
Frosting	Yogurt	

Also avoid foods that contain the following sweeteners. Remember to read the labels.

Brown sugar
Cane sugar
Corn syrup
Demerara sugar
Dextrose
Fructose
Galactose
Honey
Glucose
Maple syrup
Turbinado sugar

High Fructose Corn
  syrup
Honey
Invert Sugar
Sucrose
Lactose
Malt
Maltodextrin
Maltose
Molasses
Rice syrup

Muscovado or Barbados
  sugar
Panocha
Powdered or
Confectioner's sugar
Sugar (granulated)
Treacle
Aspartame
Splenda

The following list includes fruits that are fairly high in sugar; these should be avoided during the 1st 3 weeks of Phase 3, even though some were in Phase 2.

Grapes
Tangerines
Oranges

Pineapple
Kiwis
Bananas

Dried Fruit
Mangos

It is important to continue Part One of Phase 3 for three weeks.

Most people don't realize how vital this part is in resetting the hypothalamus. Again we are repeating ourselves but it needs to be understood; you will be establishing a new set point for your weight. By strictly following this phase of the protocol, your body will not put all the weight back on that you just lost, when you return to normal eating.

Try not to worry and focus on all the things you can't have during Phase 3. There are so many more options in this phase than there were in Phase 2.

- **The following lists contain foods you <u>can</u> eat during Phase 3.**

There are published cookbooks written specifically for Phase 3 that be found online or at your local health food store.

Low Carb Vegetables

This list is roughly arranged from lowest to highest carbohydrate counts, but all are non-starchy and generally low in carbohydrates.

Sprouts (bean, alfalfa, etc.)
Greens – lettuces, spinach, chard, etc.
Hearty Greens - collards,
  mustard greens, kale, etc.
Herbs - parsley, cilantro, basil,
  rosemary, thyme, etc.
Bok Choy
Celery
Radishes
Cabbage (or sauerkraut)
Mushrooms
Jicama
Avocado
Cucumbers (or pickles without
  added sugars)
Asparagus
Green Beans and Wax Beans
Broccoli
Cauliflower

Peppers
Summer Squash (including Zucchini)
Scallions or green onions
Bamboo Shoots
Leeks
Brussels sprouts
Snow Peas (pods)
Tomatoes
Eggplant
Artichoke Hearts
Fennel
Onions
Okra
Spaghetti Squash
Celery Root (Celeriac)
Carrots
Turnips
Water Chestnuts
Pumpkin

Eat Low Sugar Fruit.

Not everyone can have fruit in maintenance. Some people have to keep it to a couple times a week, or they gain weight.

The following list of fruit is arranged by sugar content, taking volume and weight, into account. This is not a complete list. Interestingly, the fruit lowest in sugar is some of the highest in nutritional value, including antioxidants.

Rhubarb   Grapefruit   Guava
Strawberries   Melons   Cherries
Cranberries   Apricots   Apples
Raspberries   Plums   Papaya
Blackberries   Peaches
Blueberries   Pears

Suggestions for healthy snacks

Celery with cheese or peanut   Strawberries with Brie Cheese
butter   Beef Jerky (if there is no MSG or
Apples with peanut butter   sugar)
Cottage cheese with real fruit   Plain yogurt with real fruit
Almonds   Organic trail mix
Peanuts   Fruit
Cheese sticks or slices   Stevia or Truvia as a sweetener
Berries with milk or cream

Part Two

Days 21 - 42

- **Continue weighing yourself every morning to control weight gain or loss.**

Just as you did during Part One, if your weight goes up 2 pounds, a steak day (refer to page 32) will bring the weight back down.

- **Slowly start adding starches and sugar, in small quantities, to your diet.** The key to this is slowly!

If you're gaining weight in Phase 3, consider the following:

❖ What are you eating? Does it have carbohydrates? Are you eating too much fruit? Are you eating too many nuts? Fruit and nuts make some people gain.

❖ Are you eating enough? Make sure you eat at least 1500 calories. If that much solid food scares you, or you just can't stuff that much into your body, try these tricks:

  ○ use coconut oil for cooking and in drinks and smoothies,
  ○ cook with butter
  ○ drink cream in tea and coffee
  ○ have cream with berries for pseudo ice cream.

❖ Are you eating too much?

❖ Are you ingesting any Splenda or Aspartame? Even as sugar substitutes, studies are now showing that it makes some people gain weight.

❖ Are you adding in the starches and sugars slowly enough?

❖ Are you doing a steak day when your weight goes up more than 2 pounds?

It takes about 3 weeks before the weight reached at the end of this phase becomes stable, i.e. does not show extreme fluctuations after an occasional excess.

- **Your metabolism and weight will be stabilized**

You will know you have stabilized to your weight set point, when you can eat whatever you like and either not gain, or only gain a pound or two that comes right back off. Some people in Part Two can eat pasta, pizza, and burgers on buns, sandwiches and desserts. They don't do it all at once and sometimes go back into "Part One" way eating for a day or so.

When your weight stays within a couple of pounds of weight gain or loss, you will know you are stabilized and you can move to Phase 4.

Phase 4 - (Maintenance)

Phase 4 is the lifetime maintenance of your new body.

When you successfully complete all the phases of the HCG protocol, you are ready to begin your new life as a thin, energetic, healthy person who is no longer a slave to hunger and food. Your hypothalamus will be reset and corrected from its abnormal operating state. Your metabolism will be high. Your hunger and food cravings will be low. You will no longer abnormally store fat in the abnormal secure fat reserves, but this is not the time to sit around like a couch potato and do nothing. Get moving! Set up a regular exercise schedule and stick to it. Eat healthy foods that are not full of additives and chemicals that will start to wear your body back down.

It is also important during the Maintenance Phase that you learn to relax and meditate, especially at high stressful times. Eat mindfully and learn to appreciate food and how it can help you or harm you, without letting it make you stressed. If you find yourself beginning to stress about food, step back, take a deep breath, and remember that food is only fuel. Stress generates cortisol which in turn makes your body store fat. Learning to let go of stress when it hits, will not only help you be happier but also healthier.

The following instructions are from Dr. Simeons' manuscript. They are some of his suggestions for healthy living habits.

• Eat plenty of protein throughout the day. This seems to be one of the critical keys to locking in your new weight.

• Drink one-half to one gallon of pure spring water daily.

• Walk for one hour per day.

• Eat a minimum of two apples per day.

• Eat a minimum of one grapefruit per day.

• Take one to three teaspoons of raw organic apple cider vinegar per day.

• Sleep seven to eight hours per night, ideally going to bed at approximately 10:00 p.m. and arising at 6:00 a.m.

• Eat a large breakfast.

• Eat six small meals per day.

• Finish your dinner three and one-half hours before bedtime.

• <u>On occasion</u> eat 100 grams of organic chicken, turkey, veal, beef, or fish before bedtime.

• Take digestive enzymes with food.

• Take probiotics (acidophilus) daily.

• Take a whole food supplement daily.

• Add cinnamon to food.

• Eat a big salad with lunch and dinner.

• Avoid lotions, creams, and body care products with propylene glycol or sodium laurel sulfate

• Add fiber from flax seed, oat bran, and acacia daily into your diet.

• Do yoga as often as you can.

• Do resistance exercise using weights.

Chapter 4

Frequently Asked Questions

*The real voyage of discovery
consists not in making new landscapes,
but in having new eyes.*

Marcel Proust

Frequently Asked Questions

What is HCG?

HCG stands for human chorionic gonadotrophin. HCG is produced in a specific part of the placenta called the syncytiotrophoblast during a woman's pregnancy. It is also produced by the human embryo shortly after conception; consequently, HCG is used as an indicator for pregnancy in pregnancy tests. HCG is a glycoprotein and is composed of an alpha subunit and a beta subunit. HCG is closely related to two other gonadotropins; luteinizing hormone (LH) and follicle stimulating hormone (FSH). It is also related to thyroid stimulating hormone (TSH). All three of which are glycoprotein hormones.

What is the purpose of HCG during pregnancy?

Research indicates that HCG is produced during pregnancy to help keep the corpus luteum intact. The corpus luteum is part of the ovary and is involved in the production of progesterone which is important during pregnancy. Researches also speculate that HCG boosts a woman's immune system during pregnancy.

How much HCG is produced by a woman when she is pregnant?

Blood serum levels of HCG can reach 200,000 i.u. per ml of serum during pregnancy. Consequently, one pregnancy can generate a large quantity of HCG without any detrimental effect on the woman's body.

How does HCG work in weight loss?

Dr. Simeons explained this well in his manuscript "*Pounds and Inches*". The following is taken directly from his document (found at the end of our book) except for a couple of grammatical errors we fixed. "The HCG allows your body to tap into your *body's* abnormal fat deposits (shoulder, upper arms, hips, thighs, and buttocks). In obese clients, these deposits are not usually accessible to the body until the person has gone through both his normal fat and structural fat as described above. This is the reason why no matter how much some people exercise and starve themselves they still have *problem areas that hold onto fat.*

The HCG coupled with the low calorie diet allows these abnormal fat deposits to be tapped into, released into the blood stream and used by the body similar to how a pregnant woman who is nauseous for weeks at a time typically remains relatively healthy and is additionally able to give birth to a healthy baby.

This release of fat/calories into the blood stream is also why clients taking the HCG are generally not hungry and generally have plenty of energy. The HCG actually releases 1500 - 4000 calories per day into the bloodstream. This is the ONLY reason why it is okay to be on a 500 calorie diet. Without the HCG releasing the abnormal fat and, therefore many calories into the bloodstream, the client would look haggard, by starving, and be facing excess nutritional deficiency. Most diets begin weight loss by depleting your structural fat (that fat which cushions your organs) and your normal fat reserves. However, they are slow to affect the abnormal fat which is stored in your abnormal fat deposits (shoulders, upper arms, hips, thighs, and buttocks) which seem to have only one efficient key to unlock them: HCG

Besides tapping into the abnormal fat deposits, HCG also proposes to affect your hypothalamus and your base metabolism. This protocol provides a detox and gives your entire system rest from the onslaught of food and drinks by allowing only a small amount of relatively healthy items to be processed in your body and your hypothalamus. Some experts feel this detox allows your hypothalamus to clear itself of the chemical build-up that could be preventing weight loss and re-establishes the natural functioning and hormone release of the hypothalamus."

What are the positive effects of HCG?

In addition to the weight loss and re-shaping of the body, many people report:

- Higher energy levels without any nervousness or an anxiety
- Improved sleep
- Clearer thought process
- Lower cholesterol and blood pressure while taking the HCG
- Feeling less irritable
- An overall feeling of wellness

What are the negative effects sometimes experienced while taking HCG?

Very few negative side effects have been observed. The few negative effects that have been observed include:
- Headaches during the first few days of starting HCG
- Some muscle weakness
- Constipation or diarrhea

What if I do the diet in phase 2 without the HCG?

You will still lose weight without using HCG during Phase 2. But during the diet you will be hungry and tired; most importantly, you will be losing muscle and structural fat instead of abnormal fat deposits in those problem, hard to lose areas. You will not have the dramatic reshaping of your body that the HCG brings. In short, you will not achieve the results you want.

The HCG present in the body allows your abnormal fat deposits to be released into the blood stream and burned by the body. This release of abnormal (stored) fat is why you won't be hungry during Phase 2 if you are taking HCG. The HCG actually releases 1500-4000 calories per day into the bloodstream. This is the only reason why it is okay to be on a 500 calorie diet. Without the HCG releasing the abnormal fat and, therefore, thousands of calories into the bloodstream, you would be nutritionally starved.

Do I need to be using any special make-up, lotion, soap, and deodorant during Phase 2?

Yes! You need to take out all your cosmetics, lotions, soaps, etc. and make sure that none of them list oil, anything that ends in –ose, fruits, or starches in their ingredients. If they do, you CANNOT use them during the 500 calorie phase of the diet. You need to use a deodorant that does not contain aluminum. We also suggest you do not use a liquid foundation. Try using powder mineral makeup or natural make-up lines.

How do I know if the HCG drops I'm buying are good quality drops?

Make sure the drops are manufactured in the United States by an FDA approved homeopathic manufacturer that has been distributing homeopathic remedies and natural health care products for a long enough time to have a solid, reputable track record.

Make sure the manufacturing facility is a federal and state registered pharmaceutical laboratory and that they use real human HCG.

The key to quality products is in 'hand-processing' the old fashioned way. Many modern facilities use automated machinery to process their remedies, but their manufacturer believes that the delicate matrix of the homeopathic can be damaged by the strong electromagnetic fields created by automated machinery. Hand-processing is more expensive and time-consuming, but a superior product is worth it.

If I'm using the HCG drops, how much do I need to complete Phase 2?

If your desired weight loss is 20 pounds or less, two (1 oz.) bottles of HCG are suggested. This will take you through 23 days of taking HCG; a total of 26 days in Phase 2 which is the minimum number of days Dr. Simeons recommends for Phase 2.

If your desired weight loss is 35 pounds or more, three or four (1 oz.) bottles of HCG are suggested. This will take you through 40 days of taking HCG, a total of 43 - 46 days in Phase 2. Take note that the average weight loss is about 1 pound a day. If you need to lose more than 35 pounds you will need to repeat the HCG round after 4-6 weeks of maintenance. Dr. Simeons recommends not using the HCG more than 40 days at a time as your body can build up immunity to it.

Due to the high demand for homeopathic HCG, it may benefit you to buy enough HCG to take you through the entire first round of Phase 2.

How long do I take HCG?

You will take HCG during "Phase 2" of the protocol along with a low calorie diet. The number of days you will take HCG is anywhere from 21 days to 40 days, depending on how much you want to lose. If you want to lose more than 39 pounds, you will do Phase 2 at second time but only after doing Phases 3 and 4 in between. Your body needs at least 6 weeks after ending HCG to start it again so it doesn't build up immunity to the HCG.

Does it matter what time you take it throughout the day?

As with any remedy or medication, the doses should be spread out evenly throughout the day to keep the HCG going through your system. For example, 8 am, 2 pm, and 8 pm is a well spaced schedule, taking .50 cc each time or 12 - 15 drops. You can also take HCG twice a day - morning and night, taking .75 cc each time or 18 – 22 drops each dose.

Is HCG legal to use in the US for weight loss?

Yes. You must have a prescription from a licensed physician to obtain HCG for injections. However, a homeopathic HCG formula is available over the counter or online. Again, make sure the HCG drops are good quality.

Are the homeopathic HCG drops FDA-Approved?

Homeopathic HCG is not registered with or approved by the FDA or Health Canada for weight loss. But good quality drops are made in laboratories which are in full compliance with FDA regulations governing pharmaceutical manufacturing facilities. Regular inspections of the facility should be made by the FDA ensure compliance with current Good Manufacturing Practices (cGMPs) and the Code of Federal Regulations (CFRs) for your safety.

Chapter 5

Motivational

Daily Journal Pages

Day 1　Weight _____　　　HCG

Gorge All Day

Food

Notes

Food

> "Most people never run far enough on their first wind to find out they've got a second. Give your dreams all you've got and you'll be amazed at the energy that comes out of you."
>
> *William James*

8 oz. of water	✓								
& other liquids									

48

Day 2   Weight _____   HCG

Gorge All Day

Food

> "True greatness is starting where you are, using what you have, doing what you can."
> *Arthur Ashe*

Notes

8 oz. of water	✔								
& other liquids									

Day 3   Weight _____   HCG ___

Lunch

Dinner

> **"Obstacles are what we see when we lose sight of our goal."**
>
> *Unknown*

Fruit

Notes

8 oz. of water	✔								
& other liquids									

Day 4   Weight _____   HCG ___

> "The soul is dyed the color of its thoughts. Think only on those things that are in line with your principles and can bear the light of day. The content of your character is your choice. Day by day, what you choose, what you think, and what you do is who you become. Your integrity is your destiny ... it is the light that guides your way."
>
> *Heraclitus*

Lunch

Fruit

Dinner

8 oz. of water	✔									
& other liquids										

51

Day 5   Weight _____   HCG ___

Lunch	
Dinner	
Fruit	

"Your current safe boundaries were once unknown frontiers."

Unknown

Notes	

8 oz. of water	✓									
& other liquids										

Day 6 Weight _____ HCG ___

Lunch
Dinner
Fruit

Notes

> "The world is round and the place which may seem like the end may also be the beginning."
>
> *Ivy Baker Priest*

8 oz. of water	✔									
& other liquids										

Day 7   Weight _____   HCG ____

Lunch

Fruit

Dinner

Fruit

Notes

"It's not so much that we're afraid of change or so in love with the old ways, but it's that place in between that we fear. It's like being between trapezes. It's Linus when his blanket is in the dryer. There's nothing to hold on to."

Marilyn Ferguson

8 oz. of water	✔									
& other liquids										

Day 8   Weight _____   HCG____

Lunch

Dinner
Fruit

> "Even if you're on the
> right track, you will get
> run over if you just
> sit there"
> *Unknown*

Notes

8 oz. of water	✔								
& other liquids									

Day 9   Weight _____   HCG ___

Lunch	
Dinner	

> **"Yesterday need not hold tomorrow hostage."**
>
> *Unknown*

Fruit	
Notes	

8 oz. of water	✔									
& other liquids										

Day 10   Weight _____   HCG ____

> "I learned that courage was not the absence of fear, but the triumph over it. The brave man is not he who does not feel afraid, but he who conquers that fear."
>
> *Nelson Mandela*

Lunch

Fruit

Dinner

Notes

8 oz. of water	✔								
& other liquids									

Day 11   Weight _____   HCG ____

Lunch	
Dinner	
Fruit	

Notes	

8 oz. of water	✔								
& other liquids									

Day 12   Weight _____   HCG ___

Lunch	
Dinner	
Fruit	

Notes	

"Change your thoughts and you change your world"

Norman Vincent Peale

8 oz. of water	✔									
& other liquids										

Day 13   Weight _____   HCG ____

Lunch
Fruit

Dinner
Fruit

> "Nearly every man who develops an idea works at it up to the point where it looks impossible, and then gets discouraged. That's not the place to become discouraged."

Notes

8 oz. of water	✓									
& other liquids										

Day 14   Weight _____   HCG ___

Lunch	
Dinner	
Fruit	

> "Failure?
> I never encountered it!
> All I ever met were
> temporary setbacks."
> *Unknown*

Notes	

8 oz. of water	✔								
& other liquids									

Day 15   Weight _____   HCG ____

Lunch	
Dinner	

> "The past is behind, learn from it;
> The future is ahead, prepare for it;
> The present is here,
> live in it."
>
> *Thomas Monson*

Fruit	
Notes	

8 oz. of water	✓								
& other liquids									

Day 16   Weight _____   HCG ___

> "The future is not some place we are going to, but one we are creating. The paths are not to be found, but made, and the activity of making them, changes both the maker and the destination."
>
> *William James*

Lunch

Dinner

Fruit

Notes

8 oz. of water	✔									
& other liquids										

Day 17   Weight _____   HCG ____

Lunch	
Dinner	
Fruit	

> "Today is the day you make your choices for tomorrow"
>
> *Unknown*

Notes	

8 oz. of water	✔								
& other liquids									

Day 18   Weight _____   HCG ___

Lunch	
Dinner	
Fruit	

Notes	

"Without faith and enterprise, nothing is begun. Without patience and perseverance, nothing is finished."

Unknown

8 oz. of water	✓									
& other liquids										

Day 19   Weight _____   HCG ___

Lunch	
Fruit	

Dinner

Fruit

Notes

> "Men go abroad to wonder at the heights of mountains, at the huge waves of the sea, at the long courses of the rivers, at the vast compass of the ocean, at the circular motions of the stars, and they pass by themselves without wondering."
>
> *Saint Augustine*
>
> **Don't forget how wonderful and amazing you are!**

8 oz. of water	✓									
& other liquids										

Day 20   Weight _____   HCG ___

Lunch	
Dinner	
Fruit	

> "We are what we repeatedly do. Excellence, then, is not an act but a habit"
>
> *Unknown*

Notes	

8 oz. of water	✔								
& other liquids									

Day 21   Weight _____   HCG ____

Lunch

Dinner

> **"The best thing about a bad attitude is you can change it."**
>
> *Unknown*

Fruit
Notes

8 oz. of water	✔									
& other liquids										

Day 22   Weight _____   HCG ____

> "When you get to the end of all the light you know and it's time to step into the darkness of the unknown, faith is knowing that one of two things shall happen: either you will be given something solid to stand on, or you will be taught how to fly."
>
> *Edward Teller*

Lunch

Fruit

Dinner

Notes

8 oz. of water	✔								
& other liquids									

Day 23   Weight _____   HCG ____

Lunch	
Dinner	
Fruit	

> "We do not quit playing because we grow old. We grow old because we stop playing."
>
> *Oliver Wendell Holmes*

Notes	

8 oz. of water	✔								
& other liquids									

Day 24   Weight _____   HCG ____

Lunch
Dinner
Fruit

Notes

"Your opinion of
yourself is the one that
matters most."

Unknown

8 oz. of water	✓								
& other liquids									

Day 25   Weight _____   HCG ____

Lunch	
Fruit	

Dinner	
Fruit	

Notes	

> "Obstacles are necessary for success because victory comes only after many struggles and countless defeats. Yet each struggle, each defeat, sharpens your skills and strengths, your courage and your endurance, your ability and your confidence and thus each obstacle is a comrade-in-arms forcing you to become better."
>
> *Og Mandino*

8 oz. of water	✔									
& other liquids										

Day 26   Weight _____   HCG ____

Lunch	
Dinner	
Fruit	

**Keep on swimming.
Keep on swimming.**

Dory (Finding Nemo)

Notes	

8 oz. of water	✔									
& other liquids										

Day 27   Weight _____   HCG ____

Lunch

Dinner

> "Don't limit yourself. Many people limit themselves to what they think they can do. You can go as far as your mind lets you. What you believe, you can achieve"
>
> *Mary Kay Ash*

Fruit

Notes

8 oz. of water	✔								
& other liquids									

Day 28   Weight _____   HCG ____

> "To always be intending to make a new and better life, but never finding the time to set about it, is like putting off eating, drinking and sleeping from one day to the next until you're dead."
>
> *Og Mandino*

Lunch

Fruit

Dinner

Notes

8 oz. of water	✔								
& other liquids									

Day 29 Weight _____ HCG ____

Lunch	
Dinner	
Fruit	

> "Stop worrying about
> the potholes in the road
> and celebrate the journey."
> *Barbara Hoffman*

Notes	

8 oz. of water	✔								
& other liquids									

Day 30   Weight _____   HCG ____

Lunch	
Dinner	
Fruit	

Notes

"The only way to live is to accept each minute as an unrepeatable miracle, which is exactly what it is: a miracle and unrepeatable."

Storm Jameson

8 oz. of water	✔									
& other liquids										

Day 31   Weight _____   HCG ___

Lunch
Fruit

Dinner
Fruit

> "Live your life each day, as you would climb a mountain. An occasional glance towards the summit keeps the goal in mind, but many beautiful scenes are to be observed from each new vantage point."
>
> *Harold B. Melchart*

Notes

8 oz. of water	✔								
& other liquids									

Day 32 Weight _____ HCG ___

Lunch
Dinner
Fruit

> "I don't want to get to the end of my life and find that I have just lived the length of it. I want to have lived the width of it as well."
>
> *Diane Ackerman*

Notes

8 oz. of water & other liquids	✔									

Day 33 Weight _____ HCG ____

Lunch	
Dinner	

> "Stop sitting there with your hands folded, looking on, doing nothing. Get into action and live this full and glorious life NOW. You have to do it."
>
> *Eileen Caddy*

Fruit	
Notes	

8 oz. of water	✔								
& other liquids									

Day 34　Weight _____　HCG ____

"To be willing is like being pregnant; either you are or you aren't. When you choose to be willing, you are preparing the soil, so to speak, before planting the seeds for personal growth."

John Chappelear

Lunch
Fruit

Dinner

Notes

8 oz. of water	✔								
& other liquids									

Day 35   Weight _____   HCG ____

Lunch	
Dinner	
Fruit	

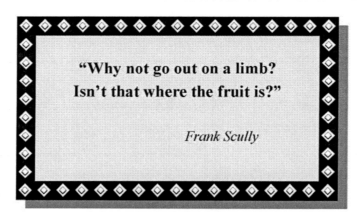

> "Why not go out on a limb?
> Isn't that where the fruit is?"
>
> *Frank Scully*

Notes	

8 oz. of water	✓								
& other liquids									

Day 36   Weight _____   HCG ____

Lunch	
Dinner	
Fruit	

Notes

"Most people have no idea of
the giant capacity we can
immediately command when
we focus all our resources on
a single area of our lives."

Anthony Robbins

8 oz. of water	✓									
& other liquids										

Day 37 Weight _____ HCG ____

Lunch

Fruit

Dinner

Fruit

Notes

> "A day merely survived is no cause for celebration. You are not here to fritter away your precious hours when you have the ability to accomplish so much by making a slight change in your routine. No more busy work. No more hiding from success. Leave time, leave space, to grow."
>
> *Og Mandino*

8 oz. of water	✔								
& other liquids									

Day 38   Weight _____   HCG ___

Lunch
Dinner
Fruit

> "The only thing that
> will stop you from
> fulfilling your dreams
> is you."
>
> *Tom Bradley*

Notes

8 oz. of water	✔								
& other liquids									

85

Day 39   Weight _____   HCG ____

Lunch

Dinner

"People often say that this or that
person has not yet found himself.
But the self is not something one finds,
it is something one creates."

Thomas Szasz

Fruit

Notes

8 oz. of water	✔									
& other liquids										

Day 40   Weight _____   HCG ____

> "We are each gifted in a unique and important way. It is our privilege and our adventure to discover our own special light."
>
> *Mary Dunbar*

Lunch

Dinner

Fruit

Notes

	✓								
8 oz. of water	✓								
& other liquids									

Day 41   Weight _____   HCG ____

Lunch	
Dinner	
Fruit	

> "It's never too late to be what you might have been."
>
> *George Eliot*

Notes	

8 oz. of water	✔								
& other liquids									

Day 42   Weight _____   HCG ____

Lunch	
Dinner	
Fruit	

Notes	

"We have to learn to be
our own best friends
because we fall too easily
into the trap of being
our own worst enemies."

Roderick Thorp

8 oz. of water	✔									
& other liquids										

Day 43 Weight _____ HCG ____

Lunch
_____

Fruit

Dinner
_____

_____

Fruit

Notes
_____

_____

8 oz. of water	✔									
& other liquids										

"The great danger for most of us is not that our aim is too high and we miss it—but that it is too low and we reach it."

Michelangelo

Day 44　Weight _____　HCG __

Lunch

Dinner

Fruit

"Look at a day when you are
supremely satisfied at the end. It's not
a day when you lounge around doing
nothing. It's when you've had
everything to do, and you've done it"

Margaret Thatcher

Notes

8 oz. of water	✓								
& other liquids									

Day 45   Weight _____ HCG ____

Lunch

Dinner

> **"A ship in harbor is safe;**
> **But that is not what ships**
> **are for."**
>
> *John A Shedd*

Fruit
Notes

8 oz. of water	✔								
& other liquids									

Additional Weight Logs and Measurement Charts

Date	Weight	Notes	Date	Weight	Notes

Weight Log at a Glance for HCG Protocol
PHASE 3

Date	Weight	Notes	Date	Weight	Notes

Date	Weight	Notes	Date	Weight	Notes

Measurements Tracking Log

Name _____

	Starting Phase 2	Midway Phase 2	End Phase 2		
Date					
Weight					
Upper chest					
Chest					
Midriff					
Waist					
Abdomen					
Hips					
Rt. Thigh					
Lft. Thigh					
Rt. Knee					
Lft. Knee					
Rt. Calf					
Lft. Calf					

Measuring Tips:

Upper Chest	at the level of under arm
Midriff	under the bust line
Waist	smallest part of the midsection
Abdomen	largest part of the midsection (below belly button & over love handles)
Thigh	at the largest part
Knee	above knee cap

In additional rows on the chart, put measurements for any extra problem areas you have, such as rolls above or below belly button, hips, mid leg, etc.

BEFORE PICTURES

AFTER PICTURES

Weight Chart for Women

Weight in pounds, based on ages 25-59 with the lowest mortality rate (height based on wearing 1" heels)

Height	Small Frame	Medium Frame	Large Frame
4'10"	92-100	97-109	105-121
4'11"	95-103	100-112	108-124
5'0"	98-106	103-115	111-127
5'1"	101-109	106-118	114-130
5'2"	104-112	109-122	117-134
5'3"	107-115	112-126	121-138
5'4"	110-119	116-131	125-152
5'5"	114-123	120-135	129-146
5'6"	118-127	124-139	133-150
5'7"	122-131	128-143	137-154
5'8"	126-136	132-147	141-159
5'9"	130-140	136-151	145-164
5'10"	133-144	140-155	149-169
5'11"	135-148	145-159	155-176
6'0"	138-151	148-162	158-179

Metropolitan Life Table

These Metropolitan Life tables became widely used for determining recommended body weights. In 1942, the tables gave "ideal body weights." In 1959, they were revised and became "desirable body weights." And in 1983, they were revised once again, this time called "height and weight tables." The weights given in the 1983 tables are heavier than the 1942 tables because, in general, heavier people live longer today.

Weight Chart for Men

Weight in pounds, based on ages 25-59 with the lowest mortality rate (height based on wearing 1" heels)

Height	Small Frame	Medium Frame	Large Frame
5'2"	128-134	131-141	138-150
5'3"	130-136	133-143	140-153
5'4"	132-138	135-145	142-156
5'5"	134-140	137-148	144-160
5'6"	136-142	139-151	146-164
5'7"	138-145	142-154	149-168
5'8"	140-148	145-157	152-172
5'9"	142-151	148-160	155-176
5'10"	144-154	151-163	158-180
5'11"	146-157	154-166	161-184
6'0"	149-160	157-170	164-188
6'1"	152-164	160-174	168-192
6'2"	155-168	164-178	172-197
6'3"	158-172	167-182	176-202
6'4"	162-176	171-187	181-207

Experts have criticized the validity of these tables for several reasons:

- Insured people tend to be healthier than uninsured people.
- Frame size was never consistently measured.
- The tables do not consider percentage of body fat or distribution, which are now known to be important factors in longevity
- Some persons were actually weighed, some were not.
- Some wore shoes and/or clothing, some did not.

The American Heart Association recommends using the 1959 tables rather than the newer tables that suggest somewhat higher weights. Our guide book shows you the 1959 tables. Some experts criticize the Metropolitan Life tables stating that they are okay for persons in their forties, but that the numbers are too heavy for younger persons and too light for older persons.

Remember that these charts are meant to give you just an estimate. The amazing thing about using the HCG protocol in your weight loss is the way your body will reshape and re-sculpt. With HCG, your body will look different at a particular weight than it may have looked otherwise, at that same weight.

Calculating Your Frame Size:

The following is the method the Metropolitan Life Insurance Company used to calculate frame size:

1. Extend your arm in front of your body bending your elbow at a ninety degree angle to your body so that your forearm is parallel to your body.
2. Keep your fingers straight and turn the inside of your wrist towards your body.
3. Place your thumb and index finger on the two prominent bones on either side of your elbow, then measure the distance between the bones with a tape measure or calipers.
4. Compare to the chart below. The chart lists elbow measurements for a medium frame - if your elbow measurement for that particular height is less than the number of inches listed, you are a small frame - if your elbow measurement for that particular height is more than the number of inches listed, then you are a large frame.

Elbow Measurements for Medium Frame			
Men	**Elbow Measurement**	**Women**	**Elbow Measurement**
5'2" - 5'3"	2-1/2" to 2-7/8"	4'10"-4'11"	2-1/4" to 2-1/2"
5'4" - 5'7"	2-5/8" to 2-7/8"	5'0" - 5'3"	2-1/4" to 2-1/2"
5'8" - 5'11"	2-3/4" to 3"	5'4" - 5'7"	2-3/8" to 2-5/8"
6'0" - 6'3"	2-3/4" to 3-1/8"	5/8" - 5'11"	2-3/8" to 2-5/8"
6'4"	2-7/8" to 3-1/4"	6'0"	2-1/2" to 2-3/4"

We want to wish you the best of luck in this weight loss adventure. We have personally had great success with the HCG protocol, along with our family members. Many clients we have coached along this journey have been able to turn their lives around. They have lost their desired weight and they've had improvement in various health issues that were a result of obesity.

We wrote this guidebook because we know it works. In our opinion, Dr. Simeons was a brilliant man in making his discoveries. We don't think he intended it to be a quick fix diet by helping you lose weight, only to go back to your old bad habits. Using the HCG protocol can give your weight loss journey a kick start; but we hope this will motivate you in all areas concerning your health and fitness. Eat healthy, have a regular exercise program, do stress relieving activities, and approach life with gusto.

Enjoy feeling fit and good about the new you; then remember to reach outside yourself and help others. A meaningful life is one spent loving, giving and doing what you can to bless someone else's life. A full life is one spent enjoying each moment and making each moment matter. Now go forward and conquer!

Carla Martell & Audrey Scott

It does little good, I decided,

to make the trip

and miss the journey.

- Max Lucado

**YOU CAN ORDER MORE BOOKS
AND HCG RECIPE BOOKS
AT:**

www.hcgskinnyme.com

The following items listed in this book, for your own use, are trademarked:

Truvia ™
Sweet Leaf ™ Liquid Flavored Stevia
Miracle Noodles ™
Konjac Flour ™
Perrier Water ™
Bragg's Amino Liquids ™
Melba Toast ™
McCormick Italian Seasoning ™
Wrights Liquid Smoke ™
George Foreman Grill ™

<u>The Original</u>

<u>Dr. Simeons' Manuscript</u>

Pounds & Inches

A NEW APPROACH TO OBESITY

BY: A.T.W. SIMEONS, M.D.

SALVATOR MUNDI INTERNATIONAL HOSPITAL
00152 - ROME
VIALE MURA GIANICOLENSI, 77

FOREWORD

This book discusses a new interpretation of the nature of obesity, and while it does not advocate yet another fancy slimming diet it does describe a method of treatment which has grown out of theoretical considerations based on clinical observation.

What I have to say is, in essence, the views distilled out of forty years of grappling with the fundamental problems of obesity, its causes, its symptoms, and its very nature. In these many years of specialized work, thousands of cases have passed through my hands and were carefully studied. Every new theory, every new method, every promising lead was considered, experimentally screened and critically evaluated as soon as it became known. But invariably the results were disappointing and lacking in uniformity.

I felt that we were merely nibbling at the fringe of a great problem, as, indeed, do most serious students of overweight. We have grown pretty sure that the tendency to accumulate abnormal fat is a very definite metabolic disorder, much as is, for instance, diabetes. Yet the localization and the nature of this disorder remained a mystery. Every new approach seemed to lead into a blind alley, and though patients were told that they are fat because they eat too much, we believed that this is neither the whole truth nor the last word in the matter.

Refusing to be side-tracked by an all too facile interpretation of obesity, I have always held that overeating is the result of the disorder, not its cause, and that we can make little headway until we can build for ourselves some sort of theoretical structure with which to explain the condition. Whether such a structure represents the truth is not important at this moment. What it must do is to give us an intellectually satisfying interpretation of what is happening in the obese body. It must also be able to withstand the onslaught of all hitherto known clinical facts and furnish a hard background against which the results of treatment can be accurately assessed.

To me this requirement seems basic, and it has always been the center of my interest. In dealing with obese patients it became a habit to register and order every clinical experience as if it were an odd looking piece of a jig-saw puzzle. And then, as in a jig saw puzzle, little clusters of fragments began to form, though they seemed to fit in nowhere. As the years passed these clusters grew bigger and started to amalgamate until, about sixteen years ago, a complete picture became dimly discernible. This picture was, and still is, dotted with gaps for which I cannot find the pieces, but I do now feel that a theoretical structure is visible as a whole.

With mounting experience, more and more facts seemed to fit snugly into the new framework, and then, when a treatment based on such speculations showed consistently satisfactory results, I was sure that some practical advance had been made, regardless of whether the theoretical interpretation of these results is correct or not.

The clinical results of the new treatment have been published in scientific journal and these reports have been generally well received by the profession, but the very nature of a scientific article does not permit the full presentation of new theoretical concepts nor is there room to discuss the finer points of technique and the reasons for observing them.

During the 16 years that have elapsed since I first published my findings, I have had many hundreds of inquiries from research institutes, doctors and patients. Hitherto I could only refer those interested to my scientific papers, though I realized that these did not contain sufficient information to enable doctors to conduct the new treatment satisfactorily. Those who tried were obliged to gain their own experience through the many trials and errors which I have long since overcome.

Doctors from all over the world have come to Italy to study the method, first hand in my clinic in the Salvator Mutidi International Hospital in Rome. For some of them the time they could spare has been too short to get a full grasp of the technique, and in any case the number of those whom I have been able to meet personally is small compared with the many requests for further detailed information which keep coming in. I have tried to keep up with these demands by correspondence, but the volume of this work has become unmanageable and that is one excuse for writing this book.

In dealing with a disorder in which the patient must take an active part in the treatment, it is, I believe, essential that he or she have an understanding of what is being done and why. Only then can there be intelligent cooperation between physician and patient. In order to avoid writing two books, one for the physician and another for the patient - a prospect which would probably have resulted in no book at all - I have tried to meet the requirements of both in a single book. This is a rather difficult enterprise in which I may not have succeeded. The expert will grumble about long-windedness while the lay-reader may occasionally have to look up an unfamiliar word in the glossary provided at the end of this manuscript.

To make the text more readable I shall be unashamedly authoritative and avoid all the hedging and tentativeness with which it is customarily to express new scientific concepts grown out of clinical experience and not as yet confirmed by clear-cut laboratory experiments. Thus, when I make what reads like a factual statement, the professional reader may have to translate into: clinical experience seems to suggest that such and such an observation might be tentatively explained by such and such a working hypothesis, requiring a vast amount of further research before the hypothesis can be considered a valid theory. If we can from the outset establish this as a mutually accepted convention, I hope to avoid being accused of speculative exuberance.

THE NATURE OF OBESITY

Obesity a Disorder

As a basis for our discussion we postulate that obesity in all its many forms is due to an abnormal functioning of some part of the body and that every ounce of abnormally accumulated fat is always the result of the same disorder of certain regulatory chanisms. Persons suffering from this particular disorder will get fat regardless of whether they eat excessively, normally or less than normal. A person who is free of the disorder will never get fat, even if he frequently overeats.

Those in whom the disorder is severe will accumulate fat very rapidly, those in whom it is moderate will gradually increase in weight and those in whom it is mild may be able to keep their excess weight stationary for long periods. In all these cases a loss of weight brought about by dieting, treatments with thyroid, appetite-reducing drugs, laxatives, violent exercise, massage, or baths is only temporary and will be rapidly regained as soon as the reducing regimen is relaxed. The reason is simply that none of these measures corrects the basic disorder.

While there are great variations in the severity of obesity, we shall consider all the different forms in both sexes and at all ages as always being due to the same disorder. Variations in form would then be partly a matter of degree, partly an inherited bodily constitution and partly the result of a secondary involvement of endocrine glands such as the pituitary, the thyroid, the adrenals or the sex glands. On the other hand, we postulate that no deficiency of any of these glands can ever directly produce the common disorder known as obesity.

If this reasoning is correct, it follows that a treatment aimed at curing the disorder must be equally effective in both sexes, at all ages and in all forms of obesity. Unless this is so, we are entitled to harbor grave doubts as to whether a given treatment corrects the underlying disorder. Moreover, any claim that the disorder has been corrected must be substantiated by the ability of the patient to eat normally of any food he pleases without regaining abnormal fat after treatment. Only if these conditions are fulfilled can we legitimately speak of curing obesity rather than of reducing weight.

Our problem thus presents itself as an enquiry into the localization and the nature of the disorder which leads to obesity. The history of this enquiry is a long series of high hopes and bitter disappointments.

The History of Obesity

There was a time, not so long ago, when obesity was considered a sign of health and prosperity in man and of beauty, amorousness and fecundity in women. This attitude probably dates back to Neolithic times, about 8000 years ago; when for the first time in the history of culture, man began to own property, domestic animals, arable land, houses, pottery and metal tools. Before that, with the possible exception of some races such as the Hottentots, obesity was almost non-existent, as it still is in all wild animals and most primitive races.

Today obesity is extremely common among all civilized races, because a disposition to the disorder can be inherited. Wherever abnormal fat was regarded as an asset, sexual selection tended to propagate the trait. It is only in very recent times that manifest obesity has lost some of its allure, though the cult of the outsize bust - always a sign of latent obesity - shows that the trend still lingers on.

The Significance of Regular Meals

In the early Neolithic times another change took place which may well account for the fact that today nearly all inherited dispositions sooner or later develop into manifest obesity. This change was the institution of regular meals.

In pre-Neolithic times, man ate only when he was hungry and only as much as he required too still the pangs of hunger. Moreover, much of his food was raw and all of it was unrefined. He roasted his meat, but he did not boil it, as he had no pots, and what little he may have grubbed from the Earth and picked from the trees, he ate as he went along.

The whole structure of man's omnivorous digestive tract is, like that of an ape, rat or pig, adjusted to the continual nibbling of tidbits. It is not suited to occasional gorging as is, for instance, the intestine of the carnivorous cat family. Thus the institution of regular meals, particularly of food rendered rapidly, placed a great burden on modern man's ability to cope with large quantities of food suddenly pouring into his system from the intestinal tract.

The institution of regular meals meant that man had to eat more than his body required at the moment of eating so as to tide him over until the next meal. Food rendered easily digestible suddenly flooded his body with nourishment of which he was in no need at the moment. Somehow, somewhere this surplus had to be stored.

Three Kinds of Fat

In the human body we can distinguish three kinds of fat. The first is the structural fat which fills the gaps between various organs, a sort of packing material. Structural fat also performs such important functions as bedding the kidneys in soft elastic tissue, protecting the coronary arteries and keeping the skin smooth and taut. It also provides the springy cushion of hard fat under the bones of the feet, without which we would be unable to walk.

The second type of fat is a normal reserve of fuel upon which the body can freely draw when the nutritional income from the intestinal tract is insufficient to meet the demand. Such normal reserves are localized all over the body. Fat is a substance which packs the highest caloric value into the smallest space so that normal reserves of fuel for muscular activity and the maintenance of body temperature can be most economically stored in this form. Both these types of fat, structural and reserve, are normal, and even if the body stocks them to capacity this can never be called obesity.

But there is a third type of fat which is entirely abnormal. It is the accumulation of such fat, and of such fat only, from which the overweight patient suffers. This abnormal fat is also a potential reserve of fuel, but unlike the normal reserves it is not available to the body in a nutritional emergency. It is, so to speak, locked away in a fixed deposit and is not kept in a current account, as are the normal reserves.

When an obese patient tries to reduce by starving himself, he will first lose his normal fat reserves. When these are exhausted he begins to burn up structural fat, and only as a last resort will the body yield its abnormal reserves, though by that time the patient usually feels so weak and hungry that the diet is abandoned. It is just for this reason that obese patients complain that when they diet they lose the wrong fat. They feel famished and tired and their face becomes drawn and haggard, but their belly, hips, thighs and upper arms show little improvement. The fat they have come to detest stays on and the fat they need to cover their bones gets less and less. Their skin wrinkles and they look old and miserable. And that is one of the most frustrating and depressing experiences a human being can have.

Injustice to the Obese

When then obese patients are accused of cheating, gluttony, lack of will power, greed and sexual complexes, the strong become indignant and decide that modern medicine is a fraud and its representatives fools, while the weak just give up the struggle in despair. In either case the result is the same: a further gain in weight, resignation to an abominable fate and the resolution at least to live tolerably the short span allotted to them - a fig for doctors and insurance companies.

Obese patients only feel physically well as long as they are stationary or gaining weight. They may feel guilty, owing to the lethargy and indolence always associated with obesity. They may feel ashamed of what they have been led to believe is a lack of control. They may feel horrified by the appearance of their nude body and the tightness of their clothes. But they have a primitive feeling of animal content which turns to misery and suffering as soon as they make a resolute attempt to reduce. For this there are sound reasons.

In the first place, more caloric energy is required to keep a large body at a certain temperature than to heat a small body. Secondly the muscular effort of moving a heavy body is greater than in the case of a light body. The muscular effort consumes calories which must be provided by food. Thus, all other factors being equal, a fat person requires more food than a lean one. One might therefore reason that if a fat person eats only the additional food his body requires he should be able to keep his weight stationary. Yet every physician who has studied obese patients under rigorously controlled conditions knows that this is not true. Many obese patients actually gain weight on a diet which is calorically deficient for their basic needs. There must thus be some other mechanism at work.

<u>Glandular Theories</u>

At one time it was thought that this mechanism might be concerned with the sex glands. Such a connection was suggested by the fact that many juvenile obese patients show an under-development of the sex organs. The middle age spread in men and the tendency of many women to put on weight in the menopause seemed to indicate a causal connection between diminishing sex function and overweight. Yet, when highly active sex hormones became available, it was found that their administration had no affect whatsoever on obesity. The sex glands could therefore not be the seat of the disorder.

The Thyroid Gland

When it was discovered that the thyroid gland controls the rate at which body-fuel is consumed, it was thought that by administering thyroid gland to obese patients their abnormal fat deposits could be burned up more rapidly. This too proved to be entirely disappointing, because as we now know, these abnormal deposits take no part in the body's energy-turnover - they are inaccessibly locked away. Thyroid medication merely forces the body to consume its normal fat reserves, which are already depleted in obese patients, and then to break down structurally essential fat without touching the abnormal deposits. In this way a patient may be brought to the brink of starvation in spite of having a hundred pounds of fat to spare. Thus any weight loss brought about by thyroid medication is always at the expense of fat of which the body is in dire need.

While the majority of obese patients have a perfectly normal thyroid gland and some even have an overactive thyroid, one also occasionally sees a case with a real thyroid deficiency. In such cases, treatment with thyroid brings about a small loss of weight, but this is not due to the loss of any abnormal fat. It is entirely the result of the elimination of a mucoid substance, called myxedema, which the body accumulates when there is a marked primary thyroid deficiency. Moreover, patients suffering only from a severe lack of thyroid hormone never become obese in the true sense. Possibly also the observation that normal persons - though not the obese - lose weight rapidly when their thyroid becomes overactive may have contributed to the false notion that thyroid deficiency and obesity are connected. Much misunderstanding about the supposed role of the thyroid gland in obesity is still met with, and it is now really high time that thyroid preparations be once and for all struck off the list of remedies for obesity. This is particularly so because giving thyroid gland to an obese patient whose thyroid is either normal or overactive, besides being useless, is decidedly dangerous.

The Pituitary Gland

The next gland to be falsely incriminated was the anterior lobe of the pituitary. This most important gland lies well protected in a bony capsule at the base of the skull. It has a vast number of functions in the body, among which is the regulation of all the other important endocrine glands. The fact that various signs of anterior pituitary deficiency are often associated with obesity raised the hope that the seat of the disorder might be in this gland. But although a large number of pituitary hormones have been isolated and many extracts of the gland prepared, not a single one or any combination of such factors proved to be of any value in the treatment of obesity. Quite recently, however, a fatmobilizing factor has been found in pituitary glands, but it is still too early to say whether this factor is destined to play a role in the treatment of obesity.

The Adrenals

Recently, a long series of brilliant discoveries concerning the working of the adrenal or suprarenal glands, small bodies which sit atop the kidneys, have created tremendous interest. This interest also turned to the problem of obesity when it was discovered that a condition which in some respects resembles a severe case of obesity - the so called Cushing's Syndrome - was caused by a glandular new-growth of the adrenals or by their excessive stimulation with ACTH, which is the pituitary hormone governing the activity of the outer rind or cortex of the adrenals.

When we learned that an abnormal stimulation of the adrenal cortex could produce signs that resemble true obesity, this knowledge furnished no practical means of treating obesity by decreasing the activity of the adrenal cortex. There is no evidence to suggest that in obesity there is any excess of adrenocortical activity; in fact, all the evidence points to the contrary. There seems to be rather a lack of adrenocortical function and a decrease in the secretion of ACTH from the anterior pituitary lobe.

So here again our search for the mechanism which produces obesity led us into a blind alley. Recently, many students of obesity have reverted to the nihilistic attitude that obesity is caused simply by overeating and that it can only be cured by under eating.

The Diencephalon or Hypothalamus

For those of us who refused to be discouraged there remained one slight hope. Buried deep down in the massive human brain there is a part which we have in common with all vertebrate animals the so-called diencephalon. It is a very primitive part of the brain and has in man been almost smothered by the huge masses of nervous tissue with which we think, reason and voluntarily move our body. The diencephalon is the part from which the central nervous system controls all the automatic animal functions of the body, such as breathing, the heart beat, digestion, sleep, sex, the urinary system, the autonomous or vegetative nervous system and via the pituitary the whole interplay of the endocrine glands.

It was therefore not unreasonable to suppose that the complex operation of storing and issuing fuel to the body might also be controlled by the diencephalon. It has long been known that the content of sugar - another form of fuel – in the blood depends on a certain nervous center in the diencephalon. When this center is destroyed in laboratory animals, they develop a condition rather similar to human stable diabetes. It has also long been known that the destruction of another diencephalic center produces a voracious appetite and a rapid gain in weight in animals which never get fat spontaneously.

The Fat-bank

Assuming that in man such a center controlling the movement of fat does exist, its function would have to be much like that of a bank. When the body assimilates from the intestinal tract more fuel than it needs at the moment, this surplus is deposited in what may be compared with a current account. Out of this account it can always be withdrawn as required. All normal fat reserves are in such a current account, and it is probable that a diencephalic center manages the deposits and withdrawals.

When now, for reasons which will be discussed later, the deposits grow rapidly while small withdrawals become more frequent, a point may be reached which goes beyond the diencephalon's banking capacity. Just as a banker might suggest to a wealthy client that instead of accumulating a large and unmanageable current account he should invest his surplus capital, the body appears to establish a fixed deposit into which all surplus funds go but from which they can no longer be withdrawn by the procedure used in a current account. In this way the diencephalic "fat-bank" frees itself from all work which goes beyond its normal banking capacity. The onset of obesity dates from the moment the diencephalon adopts this labor-saving ruse. Once a fixed deposit has been established the normal fat reserves are held at a minimum, while every available surplus is locked away in the fixed deposit and is therefore taken out of normal circulation.

Three Basic Causes of Obesity

The Inherited Factor

Assuming that there is a limit to the diencephalon's fat banking capacity, it follows that there are three basic ways in which obesity can become manifest. The first is that the fat-banking capacity is abnormally low from birth. Such a congenitally low diencephalic capacity would then represent the inherited factor in obesity. When this abnormal trait is markedly present, obesity will develop at an early age in spite of normal feeding; this could explain why among brothers and sisters eating the same food at the same table some become obese and others do not.

Other Diencephalic Disorders

The second way in which obesity can become established is the lowering of a previously normal fat-banking capacity owing to some other diencephalic disorder. It seems to be a general rule that when one of the many diencephalic centers is particularly overtaxed; it tries to increase its capacity at the expense of other centers.

In the menopause and after castration the hormones previously produced in the sex-glands no longer circulate in the body. In the presence of normally functioning sex-glands their hormones act as a brake on the secretion of the sex-gland stimulating hormones of the anterior pituitary. When this brake is removed the anterior pituitary enormously increases its output of these sex-gland stimulating hormones, though they are now no longer effective. In the absence of any response from the non-functioning or missing sex glands, there is nothing to stop the anterior pituitary from producing more and more of these hormones. This situation causes an excessive strain on the diencephalic center which controls the function of the anterior pituitary. In order to cope with this additional burden the center appears to draw more and more energy away from other centers, such as those concerned with emotional stability, the blood circulation (hot flushes) and other autonomous nervous regulations, particularly also from the not so vitally important fat-bank.

The so called stable type of diabetes involves the diencephalic blood sugar regulating center the diencephalon tries to meet this abnormal load by switching energy destined for the fat bank over to the sugar-regulating center, with the result that the fat-banking capacity is reduced to the point at which it is forced to establish a fixed deposit and thus initiate the disorder we call obesity. In this case one would have to consider the diabetes the primary cause of the obesity, but it is also possible that the process is reversed in the sense that a deficient or overworked fat-center draws energy from the sugar-center, in which case the obesity would be the cause of that type of diabetes in which the pancreas is not primarily involved. Finally, it is conceivable that in Cushing's syndrome those symptoms which resemble obesity are entirely due to the withdrawal of energy from the diencephalic fat-bank in order to make it available to the highly disturbed center which governs the anterior pituitary adrenocortical system.

Whether obesity is caused by a marked inherited deficiency of the fat-center or by some entirely different diencephalic regulatory disorder, its insurgence obviously has nothing to do with overeating and in either case obesity is certain to develop regardless of dietary restrictions. In these cases any enforced food deficit is made up from essential fat reserves and normal structural fat, much to the disadvantage of the patient's general health.

The Exhaustion of the Fat-bank

But there is still a third way in which obesity can become established, and that is when a presumably normal fat-center is suddenly (with emphasis on suddenly) called upon to deal with an enormous influx of food far in excess of momentary requirements. At first glance it does seem that here we have a straight-forward case of overeating being responsible for obesity, but on further analysis it soon becomes clear that the relation of cause and effect is not so simple. In the first place we are merely assuming that the capacity of the fat center is normal while it is possible and even probable that the only persons who have some inherited trait in this direction can become obese merely by overeating.

Secondly, in many of these cases the amount of food eaten remains the same and it is only the consumption of fuel which is suddenly decreased, as when an athlete is confined to bed for many weeks with a broken bone or when a man leading a highly active life is suddenly tied to his desk in an office and to television at home. Similarly, when a person, grown up in a cold climate, is transferred to a tropical country and continues to eat as before, he may develop obesity because in the heat far less fuel is required to maintain the normal body temperature.

When a person suffers a long period of privation, be it due to chronic illness, poverty, famine or the exigencies of war, his diencephalic regulations adjust themselves to some extent to the low food intake. When then suddenly these conditions change and he is free to eat all the food he wants, this is liable to overwhelm his fat-regulating center. During the last war (WW II) about 6000 grossly underfed Polish refugees who had spent harrowing years in Russia were transferred to a camp in India where they were well housed, given normal British army rations and some cash to buy a few extras. Within about three months, 85% were suffering from obesity.

In a person eating coarse and unrefined food, the digestion is slow and only a little nourishment at a time is assimilated from the intestinal tract. When such a person is suddenly able to obtain highly refined foods such as sugar, white flour, butter and oil these are so rapidly digested and assimilated that the rush of incoming fuel which occurs at every meal may eventually overpower the diencephalic regulatory mechanisms and thus lead to obesity. This is commonly seen in the poor man who suddenly becomes rich enough to buy the more expensive refined foods, though his total caloric intake remains the same or is even less than before.

Psychological Aspects

Much has been written about the psychological aspects of obesity. Among its many functions the diencephalon is also the seat of our primitive animal instincts, and just as in an emergency it can switch energy from one center to another, so it seems to be able to transfer pressure from one instinct to another. Thus, a lonely and unhappy person deprived of all emotional comfort and of all instinct gratification except the stilling of hunger and thirst can use these as outlets for pent up instinct pressure and so develop obesity. Yet once that has happened, no amount of psychotherapy or analysis, happiness, company or the gratification of other instincts will correct the condition.

Compulsive Eating

No end of injustice is done to obese patients by accusing them of compulsive eating, which is a form of diverted sex gratification. Most obese patients do not suffer from compulsive eating; they suffer genuine hunger - real, gnawing, torturing hunger - which has nothing whatever to do with compulsive eating. Even their sudden desire for sweets is merely the result of the experience that sweets, pastries and alcohol will most rapidly of all foods allay the pangs of hunger. This has nothing to do with diverted instincts.

On the other hand, compulsive eating does occur in some obese patients, particularly in girls in their late teens or early twenties. Fortunately from the obese patients' greater need for food, it comes on in attacks and is never associated with real hunger, a fact which is readily admitted by the patients. They only feel a feral desire to stuff. Two pounds of chocolates may be devoured in a few minutes; cold, greasy food from the refrigerator, stale bread, leftovers on stacked plates, almost anything edible is crammed down with terrifying speed and ferocity.

I have occasionally been able to watch such an attack without the patient's knowledge, and it is a frightening, ugly spectacle to behold, even if one does realize that mechanisms entirely beyond the patient's control are at work. A careful enquiry into what may have brought on such an attack almost invariably reveals that it is preceded by a strong unresolved sex-stimulation, the higher centers of the brain having blocked primitive diencephalic instinct gratification. The pressure is then let off through another primitive channel, which is oral gratification. In my experience the only thing that will cure this condition is uninhibited sex, a therapeutic procedure which is hardly ever feasible, for if it were, the patient would have adopted it without professional prompting, nor would this in any way correct the associated obesity. It would only raise new and often greater problems if used as a therapeutic measure.

Patients suffering from real compulsive eating are comparatively rare. In my practice they constitute about 1-2%. Treating them for obesity is a heartrending job. They do perfectly well between attacks, but a single bout occurring while under treatment may annul several weeks of therapy. Little wonder that such patients become discouraged. In these cases I have found that psychotherapy may make the patient fully understand the mechanism, but it does nothing to stop it. Perhaps society's growing sexual permissiveness will make compulsive eating even rarer.

Whether a patient is really suffering from compulsive eating or not is hard to decide before treatment because many obese patients think that their desire for food (to them unmotivated) is due to compulsive eating, while all the time it is merely a greater need for food. The only way to find out is to treat such patients. Those that suffer from real compulsive eating continue to have such attacks, while those who are not compulsive eaters never get an attack during treatment.

Reluctance to Lose Weight

Some patients are deeply attached to their fat and cannot bear the thought of losing it. If they are intelligent, popular and successful in spite of their handicap, this is a source of pride. Some fat girls look upon their condition as a safeguard against erotic involvements, of which they are afraid. They work out a pattern of life in which their obesity plays a determining role and then become reluctant to upset this pattern and face a new kind of life which will be entirely different after their figure has become normal and often very attractive. They fear that people will like them - or be jealous - on account of their figure rather than be attracted by their intelligence or character only. Some have a feeling that reducing means giving up an almost cherished and intimate part of them. In many of these cases psychotherapy can be helpful, as it enables these patients to see the whole situation in the full light of consciousness. An affectionate attachment to abnormal fat is usually seen in patients who became obese in childhood, but this is not necessarily so.

In all other cases the best psychotherapy can do in the usual treatment of obesity is to render the burden of hunger and never-ending dietary restrictions slightly more tolerable. Patients who have successfully established an erotic transfer to their psychiatrist are often better able to bear their suffering as a secret labor of love.

There are thus a large number of ways in which obesity can be initiated, though the disorder itself is always due to the same mechanism, an inadequacy of the diencephalic fat-center and the laying down of abnormally fixed fat deposits in abnormal places. This means that once obesity has become established, it can no more be cured by eliminating those factors which brought it on than a fire can be extinguished by removing the cause of the conflagration. Thus a discussion of the various ways in which obesity can become established is useful from a preventative point of view, but it has no bearing on the treatment of the established condition. The elimination of factors which are clearly hastening the course of the disorder may slow down its progress or even halt it, but they can never correct it.

<u>Not by Weight alone</u>

Weight alone is not a satisfactory criterion by which to judge whether a person is suffering from the disorder we call obesity or not. Every physician is familiar with the sylphlike lady who enters the consulting room and declares emphatically that she is getting horribly fat and wishes to reduce. Many an honest and sympathetic physician at once concludes that he is dealing with a "nut." If he is busy he will give her short shrift, but if he has time he will weigh her and show her tables to prove that she is actually underweight.

I have never yet seen or heard of such a lady being convinced by either procedure. The reason is that in my experience the lady is nearly always right and the doctor wrong. When such a patient is carefully examined one finds many signs of potential obesity, which is just about to become manifest as overweight. The patient distinctly feels that something is wrong with her, that a subtle change is taking place in her body, and this alarms her.

There are a number of signs and symptoms which are characteristic of obesity. In manifest obesity many and often all these signs and symptoms are present. In latent or just beginning cases some are always found, and it should be a rule that if two or more of the bodily signs are present, the case must be regarded as one that needs immediate help.

Signs and symptoms of obesity

The bodily signs may be divided into such as have developed before puberty, indicating a strong inherited factor, and those which develop at the onset of manifest disorder. Early signs are a disproportionately large size of the two upper front teeth, the first incisor, or a dimple on both sides of the sacral bone just above the buttocks. When the arms are outstretched with the palms upward, the forearms appear sharply angled outward from the upper arms. The same applies to the lower extremities. The patient cannot bring his feet together without the knees overlapping; he is, in fact, knock-kneed.

The beginning accumulation of abnormal fat shows as a little pad just below the nape of the neck, colloquially known as the Duchess' Hump. There is a triangular fatty bulge in front of the armpit when the arm is held against the body. When the skin is stretched by fat rapidly accumulating under it, it many split in the lower layers. When large and fresh, such tears are purple, but later they are transformed into white scar-tissue. Such striation, as it is called, commonly occurs on the abdomen of women during pregnancy, but in obesity it is frequently found on the breasts, the hips and occasionally on the shoulders. In many cases striation is so fine that the small white lines are only just visible. They are always a sure sign of obesity, and though this may be slight at the time of examination such patients can usually remember a period in their childhood when they were excessively chubby.

Another typical sign is a pad of fat on the insides of the knees, a spot where normal fat reserves are never stored. There may be a fold of skin over the pubic area and another fold may stretch round both sides of the chest, where a loose roll of fat can be picked up between two fingers. In the male an excessive accumulation of fat in the breasts is always indicative, while in the female the breast is usually, but not necessarily, large. Obviously excessive fat on the abdomen, the hips, thighs, upper arms, chin and shoulders are characteristic, and it is important to remember that any number of these signs may be present in persons whose weight is statistically normal; particularly if they are dieting on their own with iron determination.

Common clinical symptoms which are indicative only in their association and in the frame of the whole clinical picture are: frequent headaches, rheumatic pains without detectable bony abnormality; a feeling of laziness and lethargy, often both physical and mental and frequently associated with insomnia, the patients saying that all they want is to rest; the frightening feeling of being famished and sometimes weak with hunger two to three hours after a hearty meal and an irresistible yearning for sweets and starchy food which often overcomes the patient quite suddenly and is sometimes substituted by a desire for alcohol; constipation and a spastic or irritable colon are unusually common among the obese, and so are menstrual disorders.

Returning once more to our sylphlike lady, we can say that a combination of some of these symptoms with a few of the typical bodily signs is sufficient evidence to take her case seriously. A human figure, male or female, can only be judged in the nude; any opinion based on the dressed appearance can be quite fantastically wide off the mark, and I feel myself driven to the conclusion that apart from frankly psychotic patients such as

119

cases of anorexia nervosa; a morbid weight fixation does not exist. I have yet to see a patient who continues to complain after the figure has been rendered normal by adequate treatment.

The Emaciated Lady

I remember the case of a lady who was escorted into my consulting room while I was telephoning. She sat down in front of my desk, and when I looked up to greet her I saw the typical picture of advanced emaciation. Her dry skin hung loosely over the bones of her face, her neck was scrawny and collarbones and ribs stuck out from deep hollows. I immediately thought of cancer and decided to which of my colleagues at the hospital I would refer her. Indeed, I felt a little annoyed that my assistant had not explained to her that her case did not fall under my specialty. In answer to my query as to what I could do for her, she replied that she wanted to reduce. I tried to hide my surprise, but she must have noted a fleeting expression, for she smiled and said "I know that you think I'm mad, but just wait." With that she rose and came round to my side of the desk. Jutting out from a tiny waist she had enormous hips and thighs.

By using a technique which will presently be described, the abnormal fat on her hips was transferred to the rest of her body which had been emaciated by months of very severe dieting. At the end of a treatment lasting five weeks, she, a small woman, had lost 8 inches round her hips, while her face looked fresh and florid, the ribs were no longer visible and her weight was the same to the ounce as it had been at the first consultation.

Fat but not Obese

While a person who is statistically underweight may still be suffering from the disorder which causes obesity, it is also possible for a person to be statistically overweight without suffering from obesity. For such persons weight is no problem, as they can gain or lose at will and experience no difficulty in reducing their caloric intake. They are masters of their weight, which the obese are not. Moreover, their excess fat shows no preference for certain typical regions of the body, as does the fat in all cases of obesity. Thus, the decision whether a borderline case is really suffering from obesity or not cannot be made merely by consulting weight tables.

The Treatment Of Obesity

If obesity is always due to one very specific diencephalic deficiency, it follows that the only way to cure it is to correct this deficiency. At first this seemed an utterly hopeless undertaking. The greatest obstacle was that one could hardly hope to correct an inherited trait localized deep inside the brain, and while we did possess a number of drugs whose point of action was believed to be in the diencephalon, none of them had the slightest effect on the fat-center. There was not even a pointer showing a direction in which pharmacological research could move to find a drug that had such a specific action. The closest approach was the appetite-reducing drugs - the amphetamines----- but these cured nothing.

A Curious Observation

Mulling over this depressing situation, I remembered a rather curious observation made many years ago in India. At that time we knew very little about the function of the diencephalon, and my interest centered round the pituitary gland. Froehlich had described cases of extreme obesity and sexual underdevelopment in youths suffering from a new growth of the anterior pituitary lobe, producing what then became known as Froehlich's disease. However, it was very soon discovered that the identical syndrome, though running a less fulminating course, was quite common in patients whose pituitary gland was perfectly normal. These are the so-called "fat boys" with long, slender hands, breasts any flat-chested maiden would be proud to posses, large hips, buttocks and thighs with striation, knock-knees and underdeveloped genitals, often with undescended testicles.

It also became known that in these cases the sex organs could he developed by giving the patients injections of a substance extracted from the urine of pregnant women, it having been shown that when this substance was injected into sexually immature rats it made them precociously mature. The amount of substance which produced this effect in one rat was called one International Unit, and the purified extract was accordingly called "Human Chorionic Gonadotrophin" whereby chorionic signifies that it is produced in the placenta and gonadotropin that its action is sex gland directed.

The usual way of treating "fat boys" with underdeveloped genitals is to inject several hundred International Units twice a week. Human Chorionic

121

Gonadotrophin which we shall henceforth simply call HCG is expensive and as "fat boys" are fairly common among Indians I tried to establish the smallest effective dose. In the course of this study three interesting things emerged. The first was that when fresh pregnancy-urine from the female ward was given in quantities of about 300 cc. by retention enema, as good results could be obtained as by injecting the pure substance. The second was that small daily doses appeared to be just as effective as much larger ones given twice a week. Thirdly, and that is the observation that concerns us here, when such patients were given small daily doses they seemed to lose their ravenous appetite though they neither gained nor lost weight. Strangely enough however, their shape did change. Though they were not restricted in diet, there was a distinct decrease in the circumference of their hips.

Fat on the Move

Remembering this, it occurred to me that the change in shape could only be explained by a movement of fat away from abnormal deposits on the hips, and if that were so there was just a chance that while such fat was in transition it might be available to the body as fuel. This was easy to find out, as in that case, fat on the move would be able to replace food. It should then he possible to keep a "fat boy" on a severely restricted diet without a feeling of hunger, in spite of a rapid loss of weight. When I tried this in typical cases of Froehlich's syndrome, I found that as long as such patients were given small daily doses of HCG they could comfortably go about their usual occupations on a diet of only 500 Calories daily and lose an average of about one pound per day. It was also perfectly evident that only abnormal fat was being consumed, as there were no signs of any depletion of normal fat. Their skin remained fresh and turgid, and gradually their figures became entirely normal, nor did the daily administration of HCG appear to have any side-effects other than beneficial.

From this point it was a small step to try the same method in all other forms of obesity. It took a few hundred cases to establish beyond reasonable doubt that the mechanism operates in exactly the same way and seemingly without exception in every case of obesity. I found that, though most patients were treated in the outpatients department, gross dietary errors rarely occurred. On the contrary, most patients complained that the two meals of 250 Calories each were more than they could manage, as they continually had a feeling of just having had a large meal.

Pregnancy and Obesity

Once this trail was opened, further observations seemed to fall into line. It is, for instance, well known that during pregnancy an obese woman can very easily lose weight. She can drastically reduce her diet without feeling hunger or discomfort and lose weight without in any way harming the child in her womb. It is also surprising to what extent a woman can suffer from pregnancy-vomiting without coming to any real harm.

Pregnancy is an obese woman's one great chance to reduce her excess weight. That she so rarely makes use of this opportunity is due to the erroneous notion, usually fostered by her elder relations, that she now has "two mouths to feed" and must "keep up her strength for the coming event. All modern obstetricians know that this is nonsense and that the more superfluous fat is lost the less difficult will be the confinement, though some still hesitate to prescribe a diet sufficiently low in Calories to bring about a drastic reduction.

A woman may gain weight during pregnancy, but she never becomes obese in the strict sense of the word. Under the influence of the HCG which circulates in enormous quantities in her body during pregnancy, her diencephalic banking capacity seems to be unlimited, and abnormal fixed deposits are never formed. At confinement she is suddenly deprived of HCG, and her diencephalic fat-center reverts to its normal capacity. It is only then that the abnormally accumulated fat is locked away again in a fixed deposit. From that moment on she is suffering from obesity and is subject to all its consequences.

Pregnancy seems to be the only normal human condition in which the diencephalic fat-banking capacity is unlimited. It is only during pregnancy that fixed fat deposits can be transferred back into the normal current account and freely drawn upon to make up for any nutritional deficit. During pregnancy, every ounce of reserve fat is placed at the disposal of the growing fetus. Were this not so, an obese woman, whose normal reserves are already depleted, would have the greatest difficulties in bringing her pregnancy to full term. There is considerable evidence to suggest that it is the HCG produced in large quantities in the placenta which brings about this diencephalic change.

Though we may be able to increase the dieneephalic fat banking capacity by injecting HCG, this does not in itself affect the weight, just as transferring monetary funds from a fixed deposit into a current account does not make a man any poorer; to become poorer it is also necessary that he freely spends the money which thus becomes available. In pregnancy the needs of the growing embryo take care of this to some extent, but in the treatment of obesity there is no embryo, and so a very severe dietary restriction must take its place for the duration of treatment.

Only when the fat which is in transit under the effect of HCG is actually consumed can more fat be withdrawn from the fixed deposits. In pregnancy it would be most undesirable if the fetus were offered ample food only when there is a high influx from the intestinal tract. Ideal nutritional conditions for the fetus can only be achieved when the mother's blood is continually saturated with food, regardless of whether she eats or not, as otherwise a period of starvation might hamper the steady growth of the embryo. It seems that HCG brings about this continual saturation of the blood, which is the reason why obese patients under treatment with HCG never feel hungry in spite of their drastically reduced food intake.

The Nature of Human Chorionic Gonadotropin

HCG is never found in the human body except during pregnancy and in those rare cases in which a residue of placental tissue continues to grow in the womb in what is known as a chorionic epithelioma. It is never found in the male. The human type of chorionic gonadotrophin is found only during the pregnancy of women and the great apes. It is produced in enormous quantities, so that during certain phases of her pregnancy a woman may excrete as much as one million International Units per day in her urine - enough to render a million infantile rats precociously mature. Other mammals make use of a different hormone, which can be extracted from their blood serum but not from their urine. Their placenta differs in this and other respects from that of man and the great apes. This animal chorionic gonadotrophin is much less rapidly broken down in the human body than HCG, and it is also less suitable for the treatment of obesity.

As often happens in medicine, much confusion has been caused by giving HCG its name before its true mode of action was understood. It has been explained that gonadotrophin literally means a sex-gland directed substance or hormone, and this is quite misleading. It dates from the early days when it was first found that HCG is able to render infantile sex glands mature, whereby it was entirely overlooked that it has no stimulating effect whatsoever on normally developed and normally functioning sex-glands. No amount of HCG is ever able to increase a normal sex function; it can only improve an abnormal one and in the young hasten the onset of puberty. However, this is no direct effect. HCG acts exclusively at a diencephalic level and there brings

124

about a considerable increase in the functional capacity of all those centers which are working at maximum capacity.

The Real Gonadotrophins

Two hormones known in the female as follicle stimulating hormone (FSH) and corpus luteum stimulating hormone (LSH) are secreted by the anterior lobe of the pituitary gland. These hormones are real gonadotrophins because they directly govern the function of the ovaries. The anterior pituitary is in turn governed by the diencephalon, and so when there is an ovarian deficiency the diencephalic center concerned is hard put to correct matters by increasing the secretion from the anterior pituitary of FSH or LSH, as the case may be. When sexual deficiency is clinically present, this is a sign that the diencephalic center concerned is unable, in spite of maximal exertion, to cope with the demand for anterior pituitary stimulation. When the administration of HCG increases the functional capacity of the diencephalon, all demands can be fully satisfied and the sex deficiency is corrected.

That this is the true mechanism underlying the presumed gonadotrophic action of HCG is confirmed by the fact that when the pituitary gland of infantile rats is removed before they are given HCG, the latter has no effect on their sex-glands. HCG cannot therefore have a direct sex gland stimulating action like that of the anterior pituitary gonadotrophins, as FSH and LSH are justly called. The latter are entirely different substances from that which can be extracted from pregnancy urine and which, unfortunately, is called chorionic gonadotrophin. It would be no clumsier, and certainly far more appropriate, if HCG were henceforth called chorionic diencephalotrophin.

HCG no Sex Hormone

It cannot he sufficiently emphasized that HCG is not sex-hormone, that its action is identical in men, women, children and in those cases in which the sex-glands no longer function owing to old age or their surgical removal. The only sexual change it can bring about after puberty is an improvement of a pre-existing deficiency, but never stimulation beyond the normal. In an indirect way via the anterior pituitary, HCG regulates menstruation and facilitates conception, but it never virilizes a woman or feminizes a man. It neither makes men grow breasts nor does it interfere with their virility, though where this was deficient it may improve it. It never makes women grow a beard or develop a gruff voice. I have stressed this point only for the sake of my lay readers, because, it is our daily experience that when patients hear the word hormone they immediately jump to the conclusion that this must have something to do with the sex- sphere. They are not accustomed as we are, to think thyroid, insulin, cortisone, adrenalin etc, as hormones.

Importance and Potency of HCG

Owing to the fact that HCG has no direct action on any endocrine gland, its enormous importance in pregnancy has been overlooked and its potency underestimated. Though a pregnant woman can produce as much as one million units per day, we find that the injection of only 125 units per day is ample to reduce weight at the rate of roughly one pound per day, even in a colossus weighing 400 pounds, when associated with a 500- Calorie diet. It is no exaggeration to say that the flooding of the female body with HCG is by far the most spectacular hormonal event in pregnancy. It has an enormous protective importance for mother and child, and I even go so far as to say that no woman, and certainly not an obese one, could carry her pregnancy to term without it.

If I can be forgiven for comparing my fellow-endocrinologists with wicked Godmothers, HCG has certainly been their Cinderella, and I can only romantically hope that its extraordinary effect on abnormal fat will prove to be its Fairy Godmother.

HCG has been known for over half a century. It is the substance which Aschheim and Zondek so brilliantly used to diagnose early pregnancy out of the urine. Apart from that, the only thing it did in the experimental laboratory was to produce precocious rats, and that was not particularly stimulating to further research at a time when much more thrilling endocrinological discoveries were pouring in from all sides, sweeping, HCG into the stiller back waters.

Complicating Disorders

Some complicating disorders are often associated with obesity, and these we must briefly discuss. The most important associated disorders and the ones in which obesity seems to play a precipitating or at least an aggravating role are the following: the stable type of diabetes, gout, rheumatism and arthritis, high blood pressure and hardening of the arteries, coronary disease and cerebral hemorrhage.

Apart from the fact that they are often - though not necessarily - associated with obesity, these disorders have two things in common. In all of them, modern research is becoming more and more inclined to believe that diencephalic regulations play a dominant role in their causation. The other common factor is that they either improve or do not occur during pregnancy. In the latter respect they are joined by many other disorders not necessarily associated with obesity. Such disorders are, for instance, colitis, duodenal or gastric ulcers, certain allergies, psoriasis, loss of hair, brittle fingernails, migraine, etc.

If HCG + diet do in the obese bring about those diencephalic changes which are characteristic of pregnancy, one would expect to see an improvement in all these conditions comparable to that seen in real pregnancy. The administration of HCG does in fact do this in a remarkable way.

Diabetes
In an obese patient suffering from a fairly advanced case of stable diabetes of many years duration in which the blood sugar may range from 3-400 mg%, it is often possible to stop all anti diabetic medication after the first few days of treatment. The blood sugar continues to drop from day to day and often reaches normal values in 2-3 weeks. As in pregnancy, this phenomenon is not observed in the brittle type of diabetes, and as some cases that are predominantly stable may
have a small brittle factor in their clinical makeup, all obese diabetics have to be kept under a very careful and expert watch.

A brittle case of diabetes is primarily due to the inability of the pancreas to produce sufficient insulin, while in the stable type, diencephalic regulations seem to be of greater importance. That is possibly the reason why the stable form responds so well to the HCG method of treating obesity, whereas the brittle type does not. Obese patients are generally suffering from the stable type, but a stable type may gradually change into a brittle one, which is usually associated with a loss of weight. Thus, when an obese diabetic finds that he is losing weight without diet or treatment, he should at once have his diabetes expertly attended to. There is some evidence to suggest that the change from stable to brittle is more liable to occur in patients who are taking insulin for their stable diabetes.

Rheumatism

All rheumatic pains, even those associated with demonstrable bony lesions, improve subjectively within a few days of treatment, and often require neither cortisone nor salicylates. Again this is a well known phenomenon in pregnancy, and while under treatment with HCG + diet the effect is no less dramatic. As it does after pregnancy, the pain of deformed joints returns after treatment, but smaller doses of pain-relieving drugs seem able to control it satisfactorily after weight reduction. In any case, the HCG method makes it possible in obese arthritic patients to interrupt prolonged cortisone treatment without a recurrence of pain. This in itself is most welcome, but there is the added advantage that the treatment stimulates the secretion of ACTH in a physiological manner and that this regenerates the adrenal cortex, which is apt to suffer under prolonged cortisone treatment.

Cholesterol

The exact extent to which the blood cholesterol is involved in hardening of the arteries, high blood pressure and coronary disease is not as yet known, but it is now widely admitted that the blood cholesterol level is governed by diencephalic mechanisms. The behavior of circulating cholesterol is therefore of particular interest during the treatment of obesity with HCG. Cholesterol circulates in two forms, which we call free and esterified. Normally these fractions are present in a proportion of about 25% free to 75% esterified cholesterol, and it is the latter fraction which damages the walls of the arteries. In pregnancy this proportion is reversed and it may be taken for granted that arteriosclerosis never gets worse during pregnancy for this very reason.

To my knowledge, the only other condition in which the proportion of free to esterified cholesterol is reversed is during the treatment of obesity with

HCG + diet, when exactly the same phenomenon takes place. This seems an important indication of how closely a patient under HCG treatment resembles a pregnant woman in diencephalic behavior.

When the total amount of circulating cholesterol is normal before treatment, this absolute amount is neither significantly increased nor decreased. But when an obese patient with abnormally high cholesterol and already showing signs of arteriosclerosis is treated with HCG, his blood pressure drops and his coronary circulation seems to improve, and yet his total blood cholesterol may soar to heights never before reached.

At first this greatly alarmed us. But then we saw that the patients came to no harm even if treatment was continued and we found in follow-up examinations undertaken some months after treatment that the cholesterol was much better than it had been before treatment. As the increase is mostly in the form of the not dangerous free cholesterol, we gradually came to welcome the phenomenon. Today we believe that the rise is entirely due to the liberation of recent cholesterol deposits that have not yet undergone calcification in the arterial wall and therefore highly beneficial.

Gout
An identical behavior is found in the blood uric acid level of patients suffering from gout. Predictably such patients get an acute and often severe attack after the first few days of HCG treatment but then remain entirely free of pain, in spite of the fact that their blood uric acid often shows a marked increase which may persist for several months after treatment. Those patients who have regained their normal weight remain free of symptoms regardless of what they eat, while those that require a second course of treatment get another attack of gout as soon as the second course is initiated. We do not yet know what diencephalic mechanisms are involved in gout; possibly emotional factors play a role, and it is worth remembering that the disease does not occur in women of childbearing age. We now give 2 tablets daily of ZYLORIC to all patients who give a history of gout and have a high blood uric acid level. In this way we can completely avoid attacks during treatment.

Blood Pressure
Patients, who have brought themselves to the brink of malnutrition by exaggerated dieting, laxatives etc, often have an abnormally low blood pressure. In these cases the blood pressure rises to normal values at the

beginning of treatment and then very gradually drops, as it always does in patients with a normal blood pressure. Normal values are always regained a few days after the treatment is over. Of this lowering of the blood pressure during treatment the patients are not aware. When the blood pressure is abnormally high, and provided there are no detectable renal lesions, the pressure drops, as it usually does in pregnancy. The drop is often very rapid, so rapid in fact that it sometimes is advisable to slow down the process with pressure sustaining medication until the circulation has had a few days time to adjust itself to the new situation. On the other hand, among the thousands of cases treated, we have never seen any untoward incident which could be attributed to the rather sudden drop in high blood pressure.

When a woman suffering from high blood pressure becomes pregnant her blood pressure very soon drops, but after her confinement it may gradually rise back to its former level. Similarly, a high blood pressure present before HCG treatment tends to rise again after the treatment is over, though this is not always the case. But the former high levels are rarely reached, and we have gathered the impression that such relapses respond better to orthodox drugs such as Reserpine than before treatment.

Peptic Ulcers

In our cases of obesity with gastric or duodenal ulcers we have noticed a surprising subjective improvement in spite of a diet which would generally be considered most inappropriate for an ulcer patient. Here, too, there is a similarity with pregnancy, in which peptic ulcers hardly ever occur. However we have seen two cases with a previous history of several hemorrhages in which a bleeding occurred within 2 weeks of the end of treatment.

Psoriasis, Fingernails, Hair, Varicose Ulcers

As in pregnancy, psoriasis greatly improves during treatment but may relapse when the treatment is over. Most patients spontaneously report a marked improvement in the condition of brittle fingernails. The loss of hair not infrequently associated with obesity is temporarily arrested, though in very rare cases an increased loss of hair has been reported. I remember a case in which a patient developed a patchy baldness - so called alopecia areata - after a severe emotional shock, just before she was about to start an HCG treatment. Our dermatologist diagnosed the case as a particularly severe one, predicting that all the hair would be lost. He counseled against the reducing treatment, but in view of my previous experience and as the patient was very anxious not to postpone reducing, I discussed the matter with the dermatologist and it was agreed that, having fully acquainted the patient with the situation, the treatment should be started. During the treatment, which lasted four weeks, the further development of the bald patches was almost, if not quite, arrested; however, within a week of having finished the course of HCG, all the remaining hair fell out as predicted by the dermatologist. The interesting point is that the treatment was able to postpone this result but not to prevent it. The patient has now grown a new shock of hair of which she is justly proud.

In obese patients with large varicose ulcers we were surprised to find that these ulcers heal rapidly under treatment with HCG. We have since treated non obese patients suffering from varicose ulcers with daily injections of HCG on normal diet with equally good results.

The "Pregnant" Male

When a male patient hears that he is about to be put into a condition which in some respects resembles pregnancy, he is usually shocked and horrified. The physician must therefore carefully explain that this does not mean that he will be feminized and that HCG in no way interferes with his sex. He must be made to understand that in the interest of the propagation of the species nature provides for a perfect functioning of the regulatory headquarters in the diencephalon during pregnancy and that we are merely using this natural safeguard as a means of correcting the diencephalic disorder which is responsible for his overweight.

TECHNIQUE

Warnings

I must warn the lay reader that what follows is mainly for the treating physician and most certainly not a do-it-yourself primer. Many of the expressions used mean something entirely different to a qualified doctor than that which their common use implies, and only a physician can correctly interpret the symptoms which may arise during treatment. Any patient who thinks he can reduce by taking a few "shots" and eating less is not only sure to be disappointed but may be heading for serious trouble. The benefit the patient can derive from reading this part of the book is a fuller realization of how very important it is for him to follow to the letter his physician's instructions.

In treating obesity with the HCG + diet method we are handling what is perhaps the most complex organ in the human body. The diencephalon's functional equilibrium is delicately poised, so that whatever happens in one part has repercussions in others. In obesity this balance is out of kilter and can only be restored if the technique I am about to describe is followed implicitly. Even seemingly insignificant deviations, particularly those that at first sight seem to be an improvement, are very liable to produce most disappointing results and even annul the effect completely. For instance, if the diet is increased from 500 to 600 or 700 Calories, the loss of weight is quite unsatisfactory. If the daily dose of HCG is raised to 200 or more units daily its action often appears to be reversed, possibly because larger doses evoke diencephalic counter-regulations. On the other hand, the diencephalon is an extremely robust organ in spite of its unbelievable intricacy. From an evolutionary point of view it is one of the oldest organs in our body and its evolutionary history dates back more than 500 million years. This has tendered it extraordinarily adaptable to all natural exigencies, and that is one of the main reasons why the human species was able to evolve. What its evolution did not prepare it for were the conditions to which human culture and civilization now expose it.

History taking

When a patient first presents himself for treatment, we take a general history and note the time when the first signs of overweight were observed. We try to establish the highest weight the patient has ever had in his life (obviously excluding pregnancy), when this was, and what measures have hitherto been taken in an effort to reduce.

It has been our experience that those patients who have been taking thyroid preparations for long periods have a slightly lower average loss of weight under treatment with HCG than those who have never taken thyroid. This is even so in those patients who have been taking thyroid because they had an abnormally low basal metabolic rate. In many of these cases the low BMR is not due to any intrinsic deficiency of the thyroid gland, but rather to a lack of diencephalic stimulation of the thyroid gland via the anterior pituitary lobe. We never allow thyroid to be taken during treatment, and yet a BMR which was very low before treatment is usually found to be normal after a week or two of HCG + diet. Needless to say, this does not apply to those cases in which a thyroid deficiency has been produced by the surgical removal of a part of an overactive gland. It is also most important to ascertain whether the patient has taken diuretics (water eliminating pills) as this also decreases the weight loss under the HCG regimen.

Returning to our procedure, we next ask the patient a few questions to which he is held to reply simply with "yes" or "no". These questions are: Do you suffer from headaches? Rheumatic pains? menstrual disorders? constipation? breathlessness or exertion? swollen ankles? Do you consider yourself greedy? Do you feel the need to eat snacks between meals?

The patient then strips and is weighed and measured. The normal weight for his height, age, skeletal and muscular build is established from tables of statistical averages, whereby in women it is often necessary to make an allowance for particularly large and heavy breasts. The degree of overweight is then calculated, and from this the duration of treatment can be roughly assessed on the basis of an average loss of weight of a little less than a pound, say 300-400 grams-per injection, per day. It is a particularly interesting feature of the HCG treatment that in reasonably cooperative patients this figure is remarkably constant, regardless of sex, age and degree of overweight.

The Duration of Treatment

Patients who need to lose 15 pounds (7 kg.) or less require 26 days treatment with 23 daily injections. The extra three days are needed because all patients must continue the 500-Calorie diet for three days after the last injection. This is a very essential part of the treatment, because if they start eating normally as long as there is even a trace of HCG in their body they put on weight alarmingly at the end of the treatment. After three days when all the HCG has been eliminated this does not happen, because the blood is then no longer saturated with food and can thus accommodate an extra influx from the intestines without increasing its volume by retaining water.

We never give a treatment lasting less than 26 days, even in patients needing to lose only 5 pounds. It seems that even in the mildest cases of obesity the diencephalon requires about three weeks rest from the maximal exertion to which it has been previously subjected in order to regain fully its normal fat-banking capacity. Clinically this expresses itself, in the fact that, when in these mild cases, treatment is stopped as soon as the weight is normal, which may be achieved in a week, it is much more easily regained than after a full course of 23 injections.

As soon as such patients have lost all their abnormal superfluous fat, they at once begin to feel ravenously hungry in spite of continued injections. This is because HCG only puts abnormal fat into circulation and cannot, in the doses used, liberate normal fat deposits; indeed, it seems to prevent their consumption. As soon as their statistically normal weight is reached, these patients are put on 800-1000 Calories for the rest of the treatment.

The diet is arranged in such a way that the weight remains perfectly stationary and is thus continued for three days after the 23rd injection. Only then are the patients free to eat anything they please except sugar and starches for the next three weeks.

Such early cases are common among actresses, models, and persons who are tired of obesity, having seen its ravages in other members of their family. Film actresses frequently explain that they must weigh less than normal. With this request we flatly refuse to comply, first, because we undertake to cure a disorder, not to create a new one, and second, because it is in the nature of the HCG method that it is self limiting. It becomes completely ineffective as soon as all abnormal fat is consumed. Actresses with a slight tendency to obesity, having tried all manner of reducing methods, invariably come to the conclusion that their figure is satisfactory only when they are underweight, simply because none of these methods remove their superfluous fat deposits. When they see that under HCG their figure improves out of all proportion to the amount of weight lost, they are nearly always content to remain within their normal weight-range.

When a patient has more than 15 pounds to lose the treatment takes longer but the maximum we give in a single course is 40 injections, nor do we as a rule allow patients to lose more than 34 lbs. (15 Kg.) at a time. The treatment is stopped when either 34 lbs. have been lost or 40 injections have been given. The only exception we make is in the case of grotesquely obese patients who may be allowed to lose an additional 5-6 lbs. if this occurs before the 40 injections are up.

Immunity to HCG

The reason for limiting a course to 40 injections is that by then some patients may begin to show signs of HCG immunity. Though this phenomenon is well known, we cannot as yet define the underlying mechanism. Maybe after a certain length of time the body learns to break down and eliminate HCG very rapidly or possibly prolonged treatment leads to some sort of counter-regulation which annuls the diencephalic effect.

After 40 daily injections it takes about six weeks before this so called immunity is lost and HCG again becomes fully effective. Usually after about 40 injections patients may feel the onset of immunity as hunger increases, which was previously absent. In those comparatively rare cases in which signs of immunity develop before the full course of 40 injections has been completed-say at the 35th injection- treatment must be stopped at once, because if it is continued the patients begin to look weary and drawn, feel weak and hungry and any further loss of weight achieved is then always at the expense of normal fat. This is not only undesirable, but normal fat is also instantly regained as soon as the patient is returned to a free diet.

Patients who need only 23 injections may be injected daily, including Sundays, as they never develop immunity. In those that take 40 injections the onset of immunity can be delayed if they are given only six injections a week, leaving out Sundays or any other day they choose, provided that it is always the same day. On the days on which they do not receive the injections they usually feel a slight sensation of hunger. At first we thought that this might be purely psychological, but we found that when normal saline is injected without the patient's knowledge the same phenomenon occurs.

Menstruation

During menstruation no injections are given, but the diet is continued and causes no hardship; yet as soon as the menstruation is over, the patients become extremely hungry unless the injections are resumed at once. It is very impressive to see the suffering of a woman who has continued her diet for a day or two beyond the end of the period without coming for her injection and then to hear the next day that all hunger ceased within a few hours after the injection and to see her once again content, florid and cheerful. While on the question of menstruation it must he added that in teenage girls the period may in some rare cases be delayed and exceptionally stop altogether. If then later this is artificially induced some weight may be regained.

Further Courses

Patients requiring the loss of more than 34 lbs. must have a second or even more courses. A second course can be started after an interval of not less than six weeks, though the pause can be more than six weeks. When a third, fourth or even fifth course is necessary, the interval between courses should be made progressively longer. Between a second and third course eight weeks should elapse, between a third and fourth course twelve weeks, between a fourth and fifth course twenty weeks and between a fifth and sixth course six months. In this way it is possible to bring about a weight reduction of 100 lbs. and more if required without the least hardship to the patient.

In general, men do slightly better than women and often reach a somewhat

higher average daily loss. Very advanced cases do a little better than early ones, but it is a remarkable fact that this difference is only just statistically significant.

Conditions that must be accepted before treatment

On the basis of this data the probable duration of treatment can he calculated with considerable accuracy and this is explained to the patient. It is made clear to him that during the course of treatment he must attend the clinic daily to be weighed, injected and generally checked. All patients that live in Rome or have resident friends or relations with whom they can stay are treated as out-patients, but patients coming from abroad must stay in the hospital, as no hotel or restaurant can be relied upon to prepare the diet with sufficient accuracy. These patients have their meals, sleep, and attend the clinic in the hospital, but are otherwise free to spend their time as they please in the city and its surroundings sightseeing, bathing or theater-going.

It is also made clear that between courses the patient gets no treatment and is free to eat anything he pleases except starches and sugar during the first 3 weeks. It is impressed upon him that he will have to follow the prescribed diet to the letter and that after the first three days this will cost him no effort, as he will feel no hunger and may indeed have difficulty in getting down the 500 Calories which he will be given. If these conditions are not acceptable the case is refused, as any compromise or half measure is bound to prove utterly disappointing to patient and physician alike and is a waste of time and energy.

Though a patient can only consider himself really cured when he has been reduced to his statistically normal weight, we do not insist that he commit himself to that extent. Even a partial loss of overweight is highly beneficial, and it is our experience that once a patient has completed a first course he is so enthusiastic about the ease with which the - to him surprising - results are achieved that he almost invariably comes back for more. There certainly can be no doubt that in my clinic more time is spent on damping over-enthusiasm than on insisting that the rules of the treatment be observed.

Examining the patient

Only when agreement is reached on the points so far discussed do we proceed with the examination of the patient. A note is made of the size of the first upper incisor, of a pad of fat on the nape of the neck, at the axilla and on the inside of the knees. The presence of striation, a suprapubic fold, a thoracic fold, angulation of elbow and knee joint, breast-development in men and women, edema of the ankles and the state of genital development in the male are noted.

Wherever this seems indicated we X-ray the sella turcica, as the bony capsule which contains the pituitary gland is called, measure the basal metabolic rate, X-ray the chest and take an electrocardiogram. We do a blood-count and a sedimentation rate and estimate uric acid, cholesterol, iodine and sugar in the fasting blood.

Gain before Loss

Patients whose general condition is low, owing to excessive previous dieting, must eat to capacity for about one week before starting treatment, regardless of how much weight they may gain in the process. One cannot keep a patient comfortably on 500 Calories unless his normal fat reserves are reasonably well stocked. It is for this reason also that every case, even those that are actually gaining must eat to capacity of the most fattening food they can get down until they have had the third injection. It is a fundamental mistake to put a patient on 500 Calories as soon as the injections are started, as it seems to take about three injections before abnormally deposited fat begins to circulate and thus become available.

We distinguish between the first three injections, which we call "non-effective" as far as the loss of weight is concerned, and the subsequent injections given while the patient is dieting, which we call "effective". The average loss of weight is calculated on the number of effective injections and from the weight reached on the day of the third injection which may be well above what it was two days earlier when the first injection was given.

Most patients who have been struggling with diets for years and know how rapidly they gain if they let themselves go are very hard to convince of the absolute necessity of gorging for at least two days, and yet this must he insisted upon categorically if the further course of treatment is to run smoothly. Those patients who have to be put on forced feeding for a week before starting the injections usually gain weight rapidly - four to six pounds in 24 hours is not unusual - but after a day or two this rapid gain generally levels off. In any case, the whole gain is usually lost in the first 48 hours of dieting. It is necessary to proceed in this manner because the gain re-stocks the depleted normal reserves, whereas the subsequent loss is from the abnormal deposits only.

Patients in a satisfactory general condition and those who have not just previously restricted their diet start forced feeding on the day of the first injection. Some patents say that they can no longer overeat because their stomach has shrunk after years of restrictions. While we know that no stomach ever shrinks, we compromise by insisting that they eat frequently of highly concentrated foods such as milk chocolate, pastries with whipped cream sugar, fried meats (particularly pork), eggs and bacon, mayonnaise, bread with thick butter and jam, etc. The time and trouble spent on pressing this point upon incredulous or reluctant patients is always amply rewarded afterwards by the complete absence of those difficulties which patients who have disregarded these instructions are liable to experience.

During the two days of forced feeding from the first to the third injection - many patients are surprised that contrary to their previous experience they do not gain weight and some even lose. The explanation is that in these cases there is a compensatory flow of urine, which drains excessive water from the body. To some extent this seems to be a direct action of HCG, but it may also be due to a higher protein intake, as we know that a protein-deficient diet makes the body retain water.

Starting treatment

In menstruating women, the best time to start treatment is immediately after a period. Treatment may also be started later, but it is advisable to have at least ten days in hand before the onset of the next period. Similarly, the end of a course of HCG should never be made to coincide with menstruation. If things should happen to work out that way, it is better to give the last injection three days before the expected date of the menses so that a normal diet can he resumed at onset. Alternatively, at least three injections should be given after the period, followed by the usual three days of dieting. This rule need not be observed in such patients who have reached their normal weight before the end of treatment and are already on a higher caloric diet.

Patients who require more than the minimum of 23 injections and who therefore skip one day a week in order to postpone immunity to HCG cannot have their third injections on the day before the interval. Thus if it is decided to skip Sundays, the treatment can be started on any day of the week except Thursdays. Supposing they start on Thursday, they will have their third injection on Saturday, which is also the day on which they start their 500 Calorie diet. They would then have no injection on the second day of dieting; this exposes them to an unnecessary hardship, as without the injection they will feel particularly hungry. Of course, the difficulty can be overcome by exceptionally injecting them on the first Sunday. If this day falls between the first and second or between the second and third injection, we usually prefer to give the patient the extra day of forced feeding, which the majority rapturously enjoy.

The Diet

The 500 Calorie diet is explained on the day of the second injection to those patients who will be preparing their own food, and it is most important that the person who will actually cook is present - the wife, the mother or the cook, as the case may be. Here in Italy patients are given the following diet sheet.

139

Breakfast:	Tea or coffee in any quantity without sugar. Only one tablespoonful of milk allowed in 24 hours. Saccharin or Stevia may be used.

Lunch:

1. 100 grams of veal, beef, chicken breast, fresh white fish, lobster, crab, or shrimp. All visible fat must be carefully removed before cooking, and the meat must be weighed raw. It must be boiled or grilled without additional fat. Salmon, eel, tuna, herring, dried or pickled fish are not allowed. The chicken breast must be removed from the bird.

2. One type of vegetable only to be chosen from the following: spinach, chard, chicory, beet-greens, green salad, tomatoes, celery, fennel, onions, red radishes, cucumbers, asparagus, cabbage.

3. One breadstick (grissino) or one Melba toast.

4. An apple, orange, or a handful of strawberries or one-half grapefruit.

Dinner : The same four choices as lunch (above.)

The juice of one lemon daily is allowed for all purposes. Salt, pepper, vinegar, mustard powder, garlic, sweet basil, parsley, thyme, marjoram, etc., may be used for seasoning, but no oil, butter or dressing.

Tea, coffee, plain water, or mineral water are the only drinks allowed, but they may be taken in any quantity and at all times.

In fact, the patient should drink about 2 liters of these fluids per day. Many patients are afraid to drink so much because they fear that this may make them retain more water. This is a wrong notion as the body is more inclined to store water when the intake falls below its normal requirements.

The fruit or the breadstick may be eaten between meals instead of with lunch or dinner, but not more than four items listed for lunch and dinner may be eaten at one meal.

No medicines or cosmetics other than lipstick, eyebrow pencil and powder may be used without special permission.

Every item in the list is gone over carefully, continually stressing the point that no variations other than those listed may be introduced. All things not listed are forbidden, and the patient is assured that nothing permissible has been left out. The 100 grams of meat must he scrupulously weighed raw after all visible fat has been removed. To do this accurately the patient must have a letter-scale, as kitchen scales are not sufficiently accurate and the butcher should certainly not be relied upon. Those not uncommon patients, who feel that even so little food is too much for them, can omit anything they wish.

There is no objection to breaking up the two meals. For instance you may have a breadstick and an apple for breakfast or an orange before going to bed, provided they are deducted from the regular meals. The whole daily ration of two breadsticks or two fruits may not be eaten at the same time, nor can any item saved from the previous day be added on the following day. In the beginning patients are advised to check every meal against their diet sheet before starting to eat and not to rely on their memory. It is also worth pointing out that any attempt to observe this diet without HCG will lead to trouble in two to three days. We have had cases in which patients have proudly flaunted their dieting powers in front of their friends without mentioning the fact that they are also receiving treatment with HCG. They let their friends try the same diet, and when this proves to be a failure - as it necessarily must - the patient starts raking in unmerited kudos for superhuman willpower.

It should also be mentioned that two small apples weighing as much as one large one never the less have a higher caloric value and are therefore not allowed though there is no restriction on the size of one apple. Some people do not realize that a tangerine is not an orange and that chicken breast does not mean the breast of any other fowl, nor does it mean a wing or drumstick.

The most tiresome patients are those who start counting Calories and then come up with all manner of ingenious variations which they compile from their little books. When one has spent years of weary research trying to make a diet as attractive as possible without jeopardizing the loss of weight, culinary geniuses who are out to improve their unhappy lot are hard to take.

Making up the Calories

The diet used in conjunction with HCG must not exceed 500 Calories per day, and the way these Calories are made up is of utmost importance. For instance, if a patient drops the apple and eats an extra breadstick instead, he will not be getting more Calories but he will not lose weight. There are a number of foods, particularly fruits and vegetables, which have the same or even lower caloric values than those listed as permissible, and yet we find that they interfere with the regular loss of weight under HCG, presumably owing to the nature of their composition. Pimiento peppers, okra, artichokes and pears are examples of this.

While this diet works satisfactorily in Italy, certain modifications have to be made in other countries. For instance, American beef has almost double the caloric value of South Italian beef, which is not marbled with fat. This marbling is impossible to remove. In America, therefore, low-grade veal should be used for one meal and fish (excluding all those species such as herring, mackerel, tuna, salmon, eel, etc., which have a high fat content, and all dried, smoked or pickled fish), chicken breast, lobster, crawfish, prawns, shrimps, crabmeat or kidneys for the other meal. Where the Italian breadsticks, the so-called grissini, are not available, one Melba toast may be used instead, though they are psychologically less satisfying. A Melba toast has about the same weight as the very porous grissini which is much more to look at and to chew.

In many countries specially prepared unsweetened and low Calorie foods are freely available, and some of these can be tentatively used. When local conditions or the feeding habits of the population make changes necessary it must be borne in mind that the total daily intake must not exceed 500 Calories if the best possible results are to be obtained, that the daily ration should contain 200 grams of fat-free protein and a very small amount of starch.

Just as the daily dose of HCG is the same in all cases, so the same diet proves to be satisfactory for a small elderly lady of leisure or a hard working muscular giant. Under the effect of HCG the obese body is always able to obtain all the Calories it needs from the abnormal fat deposits, regardless of whether it uses up 1500 or 4000 per day. It must be made very clear to the patient that he is living to a far greater extent on the fat which he is losing than on what he eats.

Many patients ask why eggs are not allowed. The contents of two good sized eggs are roughly equivalent to 100 grams of meat, but fortunately the yolk contains a large amount of fat, which is undesirable. Very occasionally we allow egg - boiled, poached or raw - to patients who develop an aversion to meat, but in this case they must add the white of three eggs to the one they eat whole. In countries where cottage cheese made from skimmed milk is available 100 grams may occasionally be used instead of the meat, but no other cheeses are allowed.

Vegetarians

Strict vegetarians such as orthodox Hindus present a special problem, because milk and curds are the only animal protein they will eat. To supply them with sufficient protein of animal origin they must drink 500 cc. of skimmed milk per day, though part of this ration can be taken as curds. As far as fruit, vegetables and starch are concerned, their diet is the same as that of non-vegetarians; they cannot be allowed their usual intake of vegetable proteins from leguminous plants such as beans or from wheat or nuts, nor can they have their customary rice. In spite of these severe restrictions, their average loss is about half that of non-vegetarians, presumably owing to the sugar content of the milk.

Faulty Dieting

Few patients will take one's word for it that the slightest deviation from the diet has under HCG disastrous results as far as the weight is concerned. This extreme sensitivity has the advantage that the smallest error is immediately detectable at the daily weighing but most patients have to make the experience before they will believe it.

Persons in high official positions such as embassy personnel, politicians, senior executives, etc., who are obliged to attend social functions to which they cannot bring their meager meal must be told beforehand that an official dinner will cost them the loss of about three days treatment, however careful they are and in spite of a friendly and would-be cooperative host. We generally advise them to avoid all-round embarrassment, the almost inevitable turn of conversation to their weight problem and the outpouring of lay counsel from their table partners by not letting it be known that they are under treatment.

They should take dainty servings of everything, hide what they can under the cutlery and book the gain which may take three days to get rid of as one of the sacrifices which their profession entails. Allowing three days for their correction, such incidents do not jeopardize the treatment, provided they do not occur all too frequently in which case treatment should be postponed to a socially more peaceful season.

Vitamins and Anemia

Sooner or later most patients express a fear that they may be running out of vitamins or that the restricted diet may make them anemic. On this score the physician can confidently relieve their apprehension by explaining that every time they lose a pound of fatty tissue, which they do almost daily, only the actual fat is burned up; all the vitamins, the proteins, the blood, and the minerals which this tissue contains in abundance are fed back into the body. Actually, a low blood count not due to any serious disorder of the blood forming tissues, improves during treatment and we have never encountered a significant protein deficiency or signs of a lack of vitamins in patients who are dieting regularly.

The First Days of Treatment

On the day of the third injection it is almost routine to hear two remarks. One is: "You know, Doctor, I'm sure it's only psychological, but I already feel quite different". So common is this remark, even from very skeptical patients that we hesitate to accept the psychological interpretation. The other typical remark is: "Now that I have been allowed to eat anything I want, I can't get it down. Since yesterday I feel like a stuffed pig. Food just doesn't seem to interest me anymore, and I am longing to get on with your diet". Many patients notice that they are passing more urine and that the swelling in their ankles is less even before they start dieting.

On the day of the fourth injection most patients declare that they are feeling fine. They have usually lost two pounds or more, some say they feel a bit empty but hasten to explain that this does not amount to hunger. Some complain of a mild headache of which they have been forewarned and for which they have been given permission to take aspirin.

During the second and third day of dieting - that is, the fifth and sixth injection-these minor complaints improve while the weight continues to drop at about double the usually overall average of almost one pound per day, so that a moderately severe case may by the fourth day of dieting have lost as much as 8- 10 lbs.

It is usually at this point that a difference appears between those patients who have literally eaten to capacity during the first two days of treatment and those who have not. The former feel remarkably well; they have no hunger, nor do they feel tempted when others eat normally at the same table. They feel lighter, more clear-headed and notice a desire to move quite contrary to their previous lethargy. Those who have disregarded the advice to eat to capacity continue to have minor discomforts and do not have the same euphoric sense of well-being until about a week later. It seems that their normal fat reserves require that much more time before they are fully stocked.

Fluctuations in weight loss

After the fourth or fifth day of dieting the daily loss of weight begins to decrease to one pound or somewhat less per day, and there is a smaller urinary output. Men often continue to lose regularly at that rate, but women are more irregular in spite of faultless dieting. There may be no drop at all for two or three days and then a sudden loss which reestablishes the normal average. These fluctuations are entirely due to variations in the retention and elimination of water, which are more marked in women than in men.

The weight registered by the scale is determined by two processes not necessarily synchronized. Under the influence of HCG, fat is being extracted from the cells, in which it is stored in the fatty tissue. When these cells are empty and therefore serve no purpose, the body breaks down the cellular structure and absorbs it, but breaking up of useless cells, connective tissue, blood vessels, etc., may lag behind the process of fat-extraction. When this happens the body appears to replace some of the extracted fat with water which is retained for this purpose. As water is heavier than fat the scales may show no loss of weight, although sufficient fat has actually been consumed to make up for the deficit in the 500-Calorie diet. When then such tissue is finally broken down, the water is liberated and there is a sudden flood of urine and a marked loss of weight. This simple interpretation of what is really an extremely complex mechanism is the one we give those patients who want to know why it is that on certain days they do not lose, though they have committed no dietary error.

Patients, who have previously regularly used diuretics as a method of reducing, lose fat during the first two or three weeks of treatment which shows in their measurements, but the scale may show little or no loss because they are replacing the normal water content of their body which has been dehydrated. Diuretics should never be used for reducing.

Interruptions of Weight Loss

We distinguish four types of interruption in the regular daily loss. The first is the one that has already been mentioned in which the weight stays stationary for a day or two, and this occurs, particularly towards the end of a course, in almost every case.

The Plateau

The second type of interruption we call a "plateau". A plateau lasts 4-6 days and frequently occurs during the second half of a full course, particularly in patients that have been doing well and whose overall average of nearly a pound per effective injection has been maintained. Those who are losing more than the average all have a plateau sooner or later. A plateau always corrects, itself, but many patients who have become accustomed to a regular daily loss get unnecessarily worried and begin to fret. No amount of explanation convinces them that a plateau does not mean that they are no longer responding normally to treatment.

In such cases we consider it permissible, for purely psychological reasons, to break up the plateau. This can be done in two ways. One is a so-called "apple day". An apple-day begins at lunch and continues until just before lunch of the following day. The patients are given six large apples and are told to eat one whenever they feel the desire though six apples is the maximum allowed. During an apple-day no other food or liquids except plain water are allowed and of water they may only drink just enough to quench an uncomfortable thirst if eating an apple still leaves them thirsty. Most patients feel no need for water and are quite happy with their six apples. Needless to say, an apple-day may never be given on the day on which there is no injection. The apple-day produces a gratifying loss of weight on the following day, chiefly due to the elimination of water. This water is not regained when the patients resume their normal 500-Calorie diet at lunch, and on the following days they continue to lose weight satisfactorily.

The other way to break up a plateau is by giving a non-mercurial diuretic for one day. This is simpler for the patient but we prefer the apple-day as we sometimes find that though the diuretic is very effective on the following day it may take two to three days before the normal daily reduction is resumed, throwing the patient into a new fit of despair. It is useless to give either an apple-day or a diuretic unless the weight has been stationary for at least four days without any dietary error having been committed.

Reaching a Former Level

The third type of interruption in the regular loss of weight may last much longer - ten days to two weeks. Fortunately, it is rare and only occurs in very advanced cases, and then hardly ever during the first course of treatment. It is seen only in those patients who during some period of their lives have maintained a certain fixed degree of obesity for ten years or more and have then at some time rapidly increased beyond that weight. When then in the course of treatment the former level is reached, it may take two weeks of no loss, in spite of HCG and diet, before further reduction is normally resumed.

Menstrual Interruption

The fourth type of interruption is the one which often occurs a few days before and during the menstrual period and in some women at the time of ovulation. It must also be mentioned that when a woman becomes pregnant during treatment - and this is by no means uncommon - she at once ceases to lose weight. An unexplained arrest of reduction has on several occasions raised our suspicion before the first period was missed. If in such cases, menstruation is delayed, we stop injecting and do a precipitation test five days later. No pregnancy test should be carried out earlier than five days after the last injection, as otherwise the HCG may give a false positive result.

Oral contraceptives may be used during treatment.

Dietary Errors

Any interruption of the normal loss of weight which does not fit perfectly into one of those categories is always due to some possibly very minor dietary error. Similarly, any gain of more than 100 grams is invariably the result of some transgression or mistake, unless it happens on or about the day of ovulation or

during the three days preceding the onset of menstruation, in which case it is ignored. In all other cases the reason for the gain must be established at once.

The patient who frankly admits that he has stepped out of his regimen when told that something has gone wrong is no problem. He is always surprised at being found out, because unless he has seen this himself he will not believe that a salted almond, a couple of potato chips, a glass of tomato juice or an extra orange will bring about a definite increase in his weight on the following day.

Very often he wants to know why extra food weighing one ounce should increase his weight by six ounces. We explain this in the following way: Under the influence of HCG the blood is saturated with food and the blood volume has adapted itself so that it can only just accommodate the 500 Calories which come in from the intestinal tract in the course of the day. Any additional income, however little this may be, cannot be accommodated and the blood is therefore forced to increase its volume sufficiently to hold the extra food, which it can only do in a very diluted form. Thus it is not the weight of what is eaten that plays the determining role but rather the amount of water which the body must retain to accommodate this food.

This can be illustrated by mentioning the case of salt. In order to hold one teaspoonful of salt the body requires one liter of water, as it cannot accommodate salt in any higher concentration. Thus, if a person eats one teaspoonful of salt his weight will go up by more than two pounds as soon as this salt is absorbed from his intestine.

To this explanation many patients reply: Well, if I put on that much every time I eat a little extra, how can I hold my weight after the treatment? It must therefore be made clear that this only happens as long as they are under HCG. When treatment is over, the blood is no longer saturated and can easily accommodate extra food without having to increase its volume. Here again the professional reader will be aware that this interpretation is a simplification of an extremely intricate physiological process which actually accounts for the phenomenon.

Salt and Reducing

While we are on the subject of salt, I can take this opportunity to explain that we make no restriction in the use of salt and insist that the patients drink large quantities of water throughout the treatment. We are out to reduce abnormal fat and are not in the least interested in such illusory weight losses as can be achieved by depriving the body of salt and by desiccating it. Though we allow the free use of salt, the daily amount taken should be roughly the same, as a sudden increase will of course be followed by a corresponding increase in weight as shown by the scale. An increase in the intake of salt is one of the most common causes for an increase in weight from one day to the next. Such an increase can be ignored, provided it is accounted for. It in no way influences the regular loss of fat.

Water

Patients are usually hard to convince that the amount of water they retain has nothing to do with the amount of water they drink. When the body is forced to retain water, it will do this at all costs. If the fluid intake is insufficient to provide all the water required, the body withholds water from the kidneys and the urine becomes scanty and highly concentrated, imposing a certain strain on the kidneys. If that is insufficient, excessive water will be with-drawn from the intestinal tract, with the result that the feces become hard and dry. On the other hand if a patient drinks more than his body requires, the surplus is promptly and easily eliminated. Trying to prevent the body from retaining water by drinking less is therefore not only futile but even harmful.

Constipation

An excess of water keeps the feces soft, and that is very important in the obese, who commonly suffer from constipation and a spastic colon. While a patient is under treatment we never permit the use of any kind of laxative taken by mouth. We explain that owing to the restricted diet it is perfectly satisfactory and normal to have an evacuation of the bowel only once every three to four days and that, provided plenty of fluids are taken, this never leads to any disturbance. Only in those patients who begin to fret after four days do we allow the use of a suppository. Patients who observe this rule find that after treatment they have a perfectly normal bowel action and this delights many of them almost as much as their loss of weight.

Investigating Dietary Errors

When the reason for a slight gain in weight is not immediately evident, it is necessary to investigate further. A patient who is unaware of having committed an error or is unwilling to admit a mistake protests indignantly when told he has done something he ought not to have done. In that atmosphere no fruitful investigation can be conducted; so we calmly explain that we are not accusing him of anything but that we know for certain from our not inconsiderable experience that something has gone wrong and that we must now sit down quietly together and try and find out what it was. Once the patient realizes that it is in his own interest that he plays an active and not merely a passive role in this search, the reason for the setback is almost invariably discovered. Having been through hundreds of such sessions, we are nearly always able to distinguish the deliberate liar from the patient who is merely fooling himself or is really unaware of having erred.

Liars and Fools

When we see obese patients there are generally two of us present in order to speed up routine handling. Thus when we have to investigate a rise in weight, a glance is sufficient to make sure that we agree or disagree. If after a few questions we both feel reasonably sure that the patient is deliberately lying, we tell him that this is our opinion and warn him that unless he comes clean we may refuse further treatment. The way he reacts to this furnishes additional proof, whether we are on the right track or not, that we now very rarely make a mistake.

If the patient breaks down and confesses, we melt and are all forgiveness and treatment proceeds. Yet if such performances have to be repeated more than two or three times, we refuse further treatment. This happens in less than 1% of our cases. If the patient is stubborn and will not admit what he has been up to, we usually give him one more chance and continue treatment even though we have been unable to find the reason for his gain. In many such cases there is no repetition, and frequently the patient does then confess a few days later after he has thought things over.

The patient who is fooling himself is the one who has committed some trifling offense against the rules but who has been able to convince himself that this is of no importance and cannot possibly account for the gain in weight. Women seem particularly prone to getting themselves entangled in such delusions. On the other hand, it does frequently happen that a patient will in the midst of a conversation unthinkingly spear an olive or forget that he has already eaten his breadstick.

A mother preparing food for the family may out of sheer habit forget that she must not taste the sauce to see whether it needs more salt. Sometimes a rich maiden aunt cannot be offended by refusing a cup of tea into which she has put two teaspoons of sugar, thoughtfully remembering the patient's taste from previous occasions. Such incidents are legion and are usually confessed without hesitation, but some patients seem genuinely able to forget these lapses and remember them with a visible shock only after insistent questioning.

In these cases we go carefully over the day. Sometimes the patient has been invited to a meal or gone to a restaurant, naively believing that the food has actually been prepared exactly according to instructions. They will say: "Yes, now that I come to think of it the steak did seem a bit bigger than the one I have at home, and it did taste better; maybe there was a little fat on it, though I specially told them to cut it all away". Sometimes the breadsticks were broken and a few fragments eaten, and "Maybe they were a little more than one". It is not uncommon for patients to place too much reliance on their memory of the diet-sheet and start eating carrots, beans or peas and then to seem genuinely surprised when their attention is called to the fact that these are forbidden, as they have not been listed.

Cosmetics

When no dietary error is elicited we turn to cosmetics. Most women find it hard to believe that fats, oils, creams and ointments applied to the skin are absorbed and interfere with weight reduction by HCG just as if they had been eaten. This almost incredible sensitivity to even such very minor increases in nutritional intake is a peculiar feature of the HCG method. For instance, we find that persons who habitually handle organic fats, such as workers in beauty

parlors, masseurs, butchers, etc. never show what we consider a satisfactory loss of weight unless they can avoid fat coming into contact with their skin.

151

The point is so important that I will illustrate it with two cases. A lady who was cooperating perfectly suddenly increased half a pound. Careful questioning brought nothing to light. She had certainly made no dietary error nor had she used any kind of face cream, and she was already in the menopause. As we felt that we could trust her implicitly, we left the question suspended. Yet just as she was about to leave the consulting room she suddenly stopped, turned and snapped her fingers. "I've got it," she said. This is what had happened : She had bought herself a new set of make-up pots and bottles and, using her fingers, had transferred her large assortment of cosmetics to the new containers in anticipation of the day she would be able to use them again after her treatment.

The other case concerns a man who impressed us as being very conscientious. He was about 20 lbs. overweight but did not lose satisfactorily from the onset of treatment. Again and again we tried to find the reason but with no success, until one day he said, "I never told you this, but I have a glass eye. In fact, I have a whole set of them. I frequently change them, and every time I do that I put a special ointment in my eye socket. Do you think that could have anything to do with it?" As we thought just that, we asked him to stop using this ointment, and from that day on his weight-loss was regular.

We are particularly averse to those modern cosmetics which contain hormones, as any interference with endocrine regulations during treatment must be absolutely avoided. Many women whose skin has in the course of years become adjusted to the use of fat containing cosmetics find that their skin gets dry as soon as they stop using them. In such cases we permit the use of plain mineral oil, which has no nutritional value. On the other hand, mineral oil should not be used in preparing the food, first because of its undesirable laxative quality, and second because it absorbs some fat-soluble vitamins, which are then lost in the stool. We do permit the use of lipstick, powder and such lotions as are entirely free of fatty substances. We also allow brilliantine to be used on the hair but it must not be rubbed into the scalp. Obviously sun-tan oil is prohibited.

Many women are horrified when told that for the duration of treatment they cannot use face creams nor have facial massages. They fear that this and the loss of weight will ruin their complexion. They can be fully reassured. Under treatment normal fat is restored to the skin, which rapidly becomes fresh and turgid, making the expression much more youthful. This is a characteristic of the HCG method which is a constant source of wonder to patients who have experienced or seen in others the facial ravages produced by the usual methods of reducing. An obese woman of 70 obviously cannot expect to have her face reduced to normal without a wrinkle, but it is remarkable how youthful her face remains in spite of her age.

The Voice

Incidentally, another interesting feature of the HCG method is that it does not ruin a singing voice. The typically obese prima donna usually finds that when she tries to reduce, the timbre of her voice is liable to change, and understandably this terrifies her. Under HCG this does not happen; indeed, in many cases the voice improves and the breathing invariably does. We have had many cases of professional singers very carefully controlled by expert voice teachers, and the maestros have been so enthusiastic that they now frequently send us patients.

Other Reasons for a Gain

Apart from diet and cosmetics there can be a few other reasons for a small rise in weight. Some patients unwittingly take chewing gum, throat pastilles, vitamin pills, cough syrups etc., without realizing that the sugar or fats they contain may interfere with a regular loss of weight. Sex hormones or cortisone in its various modern forms must be avoided, though oral contraceptives are permitted. In fact the only self-medication we allow is aspirin for a headache, though headaches almost invariably disappear after a week of treatment, particularly if of the migraine type.

Occasionally we allow a sleeping tablet or a tranquilizer, but patients should be told that while under treatment they need and may get less sleep. For instance, here in Italy where it is customary to sleep during the siesta which lasts from one to four in the afternoon most patients find that though they lie down they are unable to sleep.

We encourage swimming and sun bathing during treatment, but it should be remembered that severe sunburn always produces a temporary rise in weight, evidently due to water retention. The same may be seen when a patient gets a common cold during treatment. Finally, the weight can temporarily increase - paradoxical though this may sound - after an exceptional physical exertion of long duration leading to a feeling of exhaustion. A game of tennis, a vigorous swim, a run, a ride on horseback or a round of golf do not have this effect; but a long trek, a day of skiing, rowing or cycling or dancing into the small hours usually result in a gain of weight on the following day, unless the patient is in perfect training. In patients coming from abroad, where they always use their cars, we often see this effect after a strenuous day of shopping on foot, sightseeing and visits to galleries and museums. Though the extra muscular effort involved does consume some additional Calories, this appears to be offset by the retention of water which the tired circulation cannot at once eliminate.

Appetite-reducing Drugs

We hardly ever use amphetamines, the appetite-reducing drugs such as Dexedrin, Dexamil, Preludin, etc., as there seems to be no need for them during the HCG treatment. The only time we find them useful is when a patient is, for impelling and unforeseen reasons, obliged to forego the injections for three to four days and yet wishes to continue the diet so that he need not interrupt the course.

Unforeseen Interruptions of Treatment

If an interruption of treatment lasting more than four days is necessary, the patient must increase his diet to at least 800 Calories by adding meat, eggs, cheese, and milk to his diet after the third day, as otherwise he will find himself so hungry and weak that he is unable to go about his usual occupation. If the interval lasts less than two weeks the patient can directly resume injections and the 500-Calorie diet, but if the interruption lasts longer he must again eat normally until he has had his third injection.

When a patient knows beforehand that he will have to travel and be absent for more than four days, it is always better to stop injections three days before he is due to leave so that he can have the three days of strict dieting which are necessary after the last injection at home. This saves him from the almost impossible task of having to arrange the 500 Calorie diet while en route, and he can thus enjoy a much greater dietary freedom from the day of his departure. Interruptions occurring before 20 effective injections have been given are most undesirable, because with less than that number of injections some weight is liable to be regained. After the 20th injection an unavoidable interruption is merely a loss of time.

Muscular Fatigue

Towards the end of a full course, when a good deal of fat has been rapidly lost, some patients complain that lifting a weight or climbing stairs requires a greater muscular effort than before. They feel neither breathlessness nor exhaustion but simply that their muscles have to work harder. This phenomenon, which disappears soon after the end of the treatment, is caused by the removal of abnormal fat deposited between, in, and around the muscles. The removal of this fat makes the muscles too long, and so in order to achieve a certain skeletal movement - say the bending of an arm - the muscles have to perform greater contraction than before. Within a short while the muscle adjusts itself perfectly to the new situation, but under HCG the loss of fat is so rapid that this adjustment cannot keep up with it. Patients often have to be reassured that this does not mean that they are "getting weak". This phenomenon does not occur in patients who regularly take vigorous exercise and continue to do so during treatment.

Massage

I never allow any kind of massage during treatment. It is entirely unnecessary and merely disturbs a very delicate process which is going on in the tissues. Few indeed are the masseurs and masseuses who can resist the temptation to knead and hammer abnormal fat deposits. In the course of rapid reduction it is sometimes possible to pick up a fold of skin which has not yet had time to adjust itself, as it always does under HCG, to the changed figure. This fold contains its normal subcutaneous fat and may be almost an inch thick. It is one of the main objects of the HCG treatment to keep that fat there. Patients and their masseurs do not always understand this and give this fat a working-over. I have seen such patients who were as black and blue as if they had received a sound thrashing.

In my opinion, massage, thumping, rolling, kneading, and shivering undertaken for the purpose of reducing abnormal fat can do nothing but harm. We once had the honor of treating the proprietress of a high class institution that specialized in such antics. She had the audacity to confess that she was taking our treatment to convince her clients of the efficacy of her methods, which she had found useless in her own case.

How anyone in his right mind is able to believe that fatty tissue can be shifted mechanically or be made to vanish by squeezing is beyond my comprehension. The only effect obtained is severe bruising. The torn tissue then forms scars, and these slowly contract making the fatty tissue even harder and more unyielding.

A lady once consulted us for her most ungainly legs. Large masses of fat bulged over the ankles of her tiny feet, and there were about 40 lbs. too much on her hips and thighs. We assured her that this overweight could be lost and that her ankles would markedly improve in the process. Her treatment progressed most satisfactorily but to our surprise there was no improvement in her ankles. We then discovered that she had for years been taking every kind of mechanical, electric and heat treatment for her legs and that she had made up her mind to resort to plastic surgery if we failed.

Re-examining the fat above her ankles, we found that it was unusually hard. We attributed this to the countless minor injuries inflicted by kneading. These injuries had healed but had left a tough network of connective scar-tissue in which the fat was imprisoned. Ready to try anything, she was put to bed for the remaining three weeks of her first course with her lower legs tightly strapped in unyielding bandages. Every day the pressure was increased. The combination of HCG, diet and strapping brought about a marked improvement in the shape of her ankles. At the end of her first course she returned to her home abroad. Three months later she came back for her second course. She had maintained both her weight and the improvement of her ankles. The same procedure was repeated, and after five weeks she left the hospital with a normal weight and legs that, if not exactly shapely, were at least unobtrusive. Where no such injuries of the tissues have been inflicted by inappropriate methods of treatment, these drastic measures are never necessary.

Blood Sugar

Towards the end of a course or when a patient has nearly reached his normal weight it occasionally happens that the blood sugar drops below normal, and we have even seen this in patients who had an abnormally high blood sugar before treatment. Such an attack of hypoglycemia is almost identical with the one seen in diabetics who have taken too much insulin. The attack comes on suddenly; there is the same feeling of light-headedness, weakness in the knees, trembling, and unmotivated sweating; but under HCG, hypoglycemia does not produce any feeling of hunger. All these symptoms are almost instantly relieved by taking two heaped teaspoons of sugar.

In the course of treatment the possibility of such an attack is explained to those patients who are in a phase in which a drop in blood sugar may occur. They are instructed to keep sugar or glucose sweets handy, particularly when driving a car. They are also told to watch the effect of taking sugar very carefully and report the following day. This is important, because anxious patients to whom such an attack has been explained are apt to take sugar unnecessarily, in which case it inevitably produces a gain in weight and does not dramatically relieve the symptoms for which it was taken, proving that these were not due to hypoglycemia. Some patients mistake the effects of emotional stress for hypoglycemia. When the symptoms are quickly relieved by sugar this is proof that they were indeed due to an abnormal lowering of the blood sugar, and in that case there is no increase in the weight on the following day. We always suggest that sugar be taken if the patient is in doubt.

Once such an attack has been relieved with sugar we have never seen it recur on the immediately subsequent days, and only very rarely does a patient have two such attacks separated by several days during a course of treatment. In patients who have not eaten sufficiently during the first two days of treatment we sometimes give sugar when the minor symptoms usually felt during the first three days of treatment continue beyond that time, and in some cases this has seemed to speed up the euphoria ordinarily associated with the HCG method.

The Ratio of Pounds to Inches

An interesting feature of the HCG method is that, regardless of how fat a patient is, the greatest circumference -- abdomen or hips as the case may be is reduced at a constant rate which is extraordinarily close to 1 cm. per kilogram of weight lost. At the beginning of treatment the change in measurements is somewhat greater than this, but at the end of a course it is almost invariably found that the girth is as many centimeters less as the number of kilograms by which the weight has been reduced. I have never seen this clear cut relationship in patients that try to reduce by dieting only.

Preparing the Solution

Human chorionic gonadotrophin comes on the market as a highly soluble powder which is the pure substance extracted from the urine of pregnant women. Such preparations are carefully standardized, and any brand made by a reliable pharmaceutical company is probably as good as any other. The substance should be extracted from the urine and not from the placenta, and it must of course be of human and not of animal origin. The powder is sealed in ampoules or in rubber-capped bottles in varying amounts which are stated in International Units. In this form HCG is stable; however, only such preparations should be used that have the date of manufacture and the date of expiry clearly stated on the label or package. A suitable solvent is always supplied in a separate ampoule in the same package.

Once HCG is in solution it is far less stable. It may be kept at room-temperature for two to three days, but if the solution must be kept longer it should always be refrigerated. When treating only one or two cases simultaneously, vials containing a small number of units say 1000 I.U. should be used. The 10 cc. of solvent which is supplied by the manufacturer is injected into the rubber- capped bottle containing the HCG, and the powder must dissolve instantly. Of this solution 1.25 cc. are withdrawn for each injection. One such bottle of 1000 I.U. therefore furnishes 8 injections. When more than one patient is being treated, they should not each have their own bottle but rather all be injected from the same vial and a fresh solution made when this is empty.

As we are usually treating a fair number of patients at the same time, we prefer to use vials containing 5000 units. With these the manufactures also supply 10 cc. of solvent. Of such a solution 0.25 cc. contain the 125 I.U., which is the standard dose for all cases and which should never be exceeded. This small amount is awkward to handle accurately (it requires an insulin syringe) and is wasteful, because there is a loss of solution in the nozzle of the syringe and in the needle. We therefore prefer a higher dilution, which we prepare in the following way: The solvent supplied is injected into the rubber capped bottle containing the 5000 I.U. As these bottles are too small to hold more solvent, we withdraw 5 cc., inject it into an empty rubber-capped bottle and add 5 cc. of normal saline to each bottle. This gives us 10 cc. of solution in each bottle, and of this solution 0.5 cc. contains 125 I.U. This amount is convenient to inject with an ordinary syringe.

Injecting

HCG produces little or no tissue-reaction, it is completely painless and in the many thousands of injections we have given we have never seen an inflammatory or suppurative reaction at the site of the injection.

One should avoid leaving a vacuum in the bottle after preparing the solution or after withdrawal of the amount required for the injections as otherwise alcohol used for sterilizing a frequently perforated rubber cap might be drawn into the solution. When sharp needles are used, it sometimes happens that a little bit of rubber is punched out of the rubber cap and can be seen as a small black speck floating in the solution. As these bits of rubber are heavier than the solution they rapidly settle out, and it is thus easy to avoid drawing them into the syringe.

We use very fine needles that are two inches long and inject deep intragluteally in the outer upper quadrant of the buttocks. The injection should if possible not be given into the superficial fat layers, which in very obese patients must be compressed so as to enable the needle to reach the muscle. Obviously needles and syringes must be carefully washed, sterilized and handled aseptically. It is also important that the daily injection should be given at intervals as close to 24 hours as possible. Any attempt to economize in time by giving larger doses at longer intervals is doomed to produce less satisfactory results.

There are hardly any contraindications to the HCG method. Treatment can be continued in the presence of abscesses, suppuration, large infected wounds and major fractures. Surgery and general anesthesia are no reason to stop and we have given treatment during a severe attack of malaria. Acne or boils are no contraindication; the former usually clears up, and furunculosis comes to an end. Thrombophlebitis is no contraindication, and we have treated several obese patients with HCG and the 500-Calorie diet while suffering from this condition. Our impression has been that in obese patients the phlebitis does rather better and certainly no worse than under the usual treatment alone. This also applies to patients suffering from varicose ulcers which tend to heal rapidly.

Fibroids

While uterine fibroids seem to be in no way affected by HCG in the doses we use, we have found that very large, externally palpable uterine myomas are apt to give trouble. We are convinced that this is entirely due to the rather sudden disappearance of fat from the pelvic bed upon which they rest and that it is the weight of the tumor pressing on the underlying tissues which accounts for the discomfort or pain which may arise during treatment. While we disregard even fair-sized or multiple myomas, we insist that very large ones be operated before treatment. We have had patients present themselves for reducing fat from their abdomen that showed no signs of obesity, but had a large abdominal tumor.

Gallstones

Small stones in the gall bladder may in patients who have recently had typical colic cause more frequent colic under treatment with HCG. This may be due to the almost complete absence of fat from the diet, which prevents the normal emptying of the gall bladder. Before undertaking treatment we explain to such patients that there is a risk of more frequent and possibly severe symptoms and that it may become necessary to operate. If they are prepared to take this risk and provided they agree to undergo an operation if we consider this imperative, we proceed with treatment, as after weight reduction with HCG the operative risk is considerably reduced in an obese patient. In such cases we always give a drug which stimulates the flow of bile, and in the majority of cases nothing untoward happens. On the other hand, we have looked for and not found any evidence to suggest that the HCG treatment leads to the formation of gallstones as pregnancy sometimes does.

The Heart

Disorders of the heart are not as a rule contraindications. In fact, the removal of abnormal fat - particularly from the heart-muscle and from the surrounding of the coronary arteries - can only be beneficial in cases of myocardial weakness, and many such patients are referred to us by cardiologists. Within the first week of treatment all patients - not only heart cases - remark that they have lost much of their breathlessness.

Coronary Occlusion

In obese patients who have recently survived a coronary occlusion, we adopt the following procedure in collaboration with the cardiologist. We wait until no further electrocardiographic changes have occurred for a period of three months. Routine treatment is then started under careful control and it is usual to find a further electrocardiographic improvement of a condition which was previously stationary.

In the thousands of cases we have treated we have not once seen any sort of coronary incident occur during or shortly after treatment. The same applies to cerebral vascular accidents. Nor have we ever seen a case of thrombosis of any sort develop during treatment, even though a high blood pressure is rapidly lowered. In this respect, too, the HCG treatment resembles pregnancy.

Teeth and Vitamins

Patients whose teeth are in poor repair sometimes get more trouble under prolonged treatment, just as may occur in pregnancy. In such cases we do allow calcium and vitamin D, though not in an oily solution. The only other vitamin we permit is vitamin C, which we use in large doses combined with an antihistamine at the onset of a common cold. There is no objection to the use of an antibiotic if this is required, for instance by the dentist. In cases of bronchial asthma and hay fever we have occasionally resorted to cortisone during treatment and find that triamcinolone is the least likely to interfere with the loss of weight, but many asthmatics improve with HCG alone.

Alcohol

Obese heavy drinkers, even those bordering on alcoholism, often do surprisingly well under HCG and it is exceptional for them to take a drink while under treatment. When they do, they find that a relatively small quantity of alcohol produces intoxication. Such patients say that they do not feel the need to drink. This may in part be due to the euphoria which the treatment produces and in part to the complete absence of the need for quick sustenance from which most obese patients suffer.

Though we have had a few cases that have continued abstinence long after treatment, others relapse as soon as they are back on a normal diet. We have a few "regular customers" who, having once been reduced to their normal weight, start to drink again though watching their weight. Then after some months they purposely overeat in order to gain sufficient weight for another course of HCG which temporarily gets them out of their drinking routine. We do not particularly welcome such cases, but we see no reason for refusing their request.

Tuberculosis

It is interesting that obese patients suffering from inactive pulmonary tuberculosis can be safely treated. We have under very careful control treated patients as early as three months after they were pronounced inactive and have never seen a relapse occur during or shortly after treatment. In fact, we only have one case on our records in which active tuberculosis developed in a young man about one year after a treatment which had lasted three weeks. Earlier X-rays showed a calcified spot from a childhood infection which had not produced clinical symptoms. There was a family history of tuberculosis, and his illness started under adverse conditions which certainly had nothing to do with the treatment. Residual calcifications from an early infection are exceedingly common, and we never consider them a contraindication to treatment.

The Painful Heel

In obese patients who have been trying desperately to keep their weight down by severe dieting, a curious symptom sometimes occurs. They complain of an unbearable pain in their heels which they feel only while standing or walking. As soon as they take the weight off their heels the pain ceases. These cases are the bane of the rheumatologists and orthopedic surgeons who have treated them before they come to us. All the usual investigations are entirely negative, and there is not the slightest response to anti- rheumatic medication or physiotherapy. The pain may be so severe that the patients are obliged to give up their occupation, and they are not infrequently labeled as a case of hysteria. When their heels are carefully examined one finds that the sole is softer than normal and that the heel bone - the calcaneus - can be distinctly felt, which is not the case in a normal foot.

We interpret the condition as a lack of the hard fatty pad on which the calcaneus rests and which protects both the bone and the skin of the sole from pressure. This fat is like a springy cushion which carries the weight of the body. Standing on a heel in which this fat is missing or reduced must obviously be very painful. In their efforts to keep their weight down, these patients have consumed this normal structural fat.

Those patients who have a normal or subnormal weight while showing the typically obese fat deposits are made to eat to capacity, often much against their will, for one week. They gain weight rapidly but there is no improvement in the painful heels. They are then started on the routine HCG treatment. Overweight patients are treated immediately. In both cases the pain completely disappears in 10-20 days of dieting, usually around the 15th day of treatment, and so far no case has had a relapse though we have been able to follow up such patients for years.

We are particularly interested in these cases, as they furnish further proof of the contention that HCG + 500 Calories not only removes abnormal fat but actually permits normal fat to be replaced, in spite of the deficient food intake. It is certainly not so that the mere loss of weight reduces the pain, because it frequently disappears before the weight the patient had prior to the period of forced feeding is reached.

The Skeptical Patient

Any doctor who starts using the HCG method for the first time will have considerable difficulty, particularly if he himself is not fully convinced, in making patients believe that they will not feel hungry on 500 Calories and that their face will not collapse. New patients always anticipate the phenomena they know so well from previous treatments and diets and are incredulous when told that these will not occur. We overcome all this by letting new patients spend a little time in the waiting room with older hands, which can always be relied upon to allay these fears with evangelistic zeal, often demonstrating the finer points on their own body.

A waiting-room filled with obese patients who congregate daily is a sort of group therapy. They compare notes and pop back into the waiting room after the consultation to announce the score of the last 24 hours to an enthralled audience. They cross-check on their diets and sometimes confess sins which they try to hide from us, usually with the result that the patient in whom they have confided palpitatingly tattles the whole disgraceful story to us with a "But don't let her know I told you."

Concluding a Course

When the three days of dieting after the last injection are over, the patients are told that they may now eat anything they please, except sugar and starch provided they faithfully observe one simple rule. This rule is that they must have their own portable bathroom-scale always at hand, particularly while traveling. They must without fail weigh themselves every morning as they get out of bed, having first emptied their bladder. If they are in the habit of having breakfast in bed, they must weigh before breakfast.

It takes about 3 weeks before the weight reached at the end of the treatment becomes stable, i.e. does not show violent fluctuations after an occasional excess. During this period patients must realize that the so-called carbohydrates, that are sugar, rice, bread, potatoes, pastries, etc, are by far the most dangerous. If no carbohydrates whatsoever are eaten, fats can be indulged in somewhat more liberally and even small quantities of alcohol, such as a glass of wine with meals, does no harm, but as soon as fats and starch are combined things are very liable to get out of hand. This has to be observed very carefully during the first 3 weeks after the treatment is ended otherwise disappointments are almost sure to occur.

Skipping a Meal

As long as their weight stays within two pounds of the weight reached on the day of the last injection, patients should take no notice of any increase but the moment the scale goes beyond two pounds, even if this is only a few ounces, they must on that same day entirely skip breakfast and lunch but take plenty to drink. In the evening they must eat a huge steak with only an apple or a raw tomato. Of course this rule applies only to the morning weight. Ex-obese patients should never check their weight during the day, as there may be wide fluctuations and these are merely alarming and confusing.

It is of utmost importance that the meal is skipped on the same day as the scale registers an increase of more than two pounds and that missing the meals is not postponed until the following day. If a meal is skipped on the day in which a gain is registered in the morning this brings about an immediate drop of often over a pound. But if the skipping of the meal - and skipping means literally skipping, not just having a light meal - is postponed the phenomenon does not occur and several days of strict dieting may be necessary to correct the situation.

Most patients hardly ever need to skip a meal. If they have eaten a heavy lunch they feel no desire to eat their dinner, and in this case no increase takes place. If they keep their weight at the point reached at the end of the treatment, even a heavy dinner does not bring about an increase of two pounds on the next morning and does not therefore call for any special measures. Most patients are surprised how small their appetite has become and yet how much they can eat without gaining weight. They no longer suffer from an abnormal appetite and feel satisfied with much less food than before. In fact, they are usually disappointed that they cannot manage their first normal meal, which they have been planning for weeks.

Losing more Weight

An ex-patient should never gain more than two pounds without immediately correcting this, but it is equally undesirable that more than two lbs. be lost after treatment, because a greater loss is always achieved at the expense of normal fat. Any normal fat that is lost is invariably regained as soon as more food is taken, and it often happens that this rebound overshoots the upper two lbs. Limit.

Trouble after Treatment

Two difficulties may be encountered in the immediate post-treatment period. When a patient has consumed all his abnormal fat or, when after a full course, the injection has temporarily lost its efficacy owing to the body having gradually evolved a counter regulation, the patient at once begins to feel much hungrier and even weak. In spite of repeated warnings, some over-enthusiastic patients do not report this. However, in about two days the fact that they are being undernourished becomes visible in their faces, and treatment is then stopped at once. In such cases - and only in such cases - we allow a very slight increase in the diet, such as an extra apple, 150 grams of meat or two or three extra breadsticks during the three days of dieting after the last injection.

When abnormal fat is no longer being put into circulation either because it has been consumed or because immunity has set in, this is always felt by the patient as sudden, intolerable and constant hunger. In this sense, the HCG method is completely self-limiting. With HCG it is impossible to reduce a patient, however enthusiastic, beyond his normal weight. As soon as no more abnormal fat is being issued, the body starts consuming normal fat, and this is always regained as soon as ordinary feeding is resumed. The patient then finds that the 2-3 lbs. he has lost during the last days of treatment are immediately regained. A meal is skipped and maybe a pound is lost. The next day this pound is regained, in spite of a careful watch over the food intake. In a few days a tearful patient is back in the consulting room, convinced that her case is a failure.

All that is happening is that the essential fat lost at the end of the treatment, owing to the patient's reluctance to report a much greater hunger, is being replaced. The weight at which such a patient must stabilize thus lies 2-3 lbs. higher than the weight reached at the end of the treatment. Once this higher basic level is established, further difficulties in controlling the weight at the new point of stabilization hardly arise.

Beware of Over-enthusiasm

The other trouble which is frequently encountered immediately after treatment is again due to over-enthusiasm. Some patients cannot believe that they can eat fairly normally without regaining weight. They disregard the advice to eat anything they please except sugar and starch and want to play safe. They try more or less to continue the 500-Calorie diet on which they felt so well during treatment and make only minor variations, such as replacing the meat with an egg, cheese, or a glass of milk. To their horror they find that in spite of this bravura, their weight goes up. So, following instructions, they skip one meager lunch and at night eat only a little salad and drink a pot of unsweetened tea, becoming increasingly hungry and weak. The next morning they find that they have increased yet another pound. They feel terrible, and even the dreaded swelling of their ankles is back. Normally we check our patients one week after they have been eating freely, but these cases return in a few days. Either their eyes are filled with tears or they angrily imply that when we told them to eat normally we were just fooling them.

Protein deficiency

Here too, the explanation is quite simple. During treatment the patient has been only just above the verge of protein deficiency and has had the advantage of protein being fed back into his system from the breakdown of fatty tissue. Once the treatment is over there is no more HCG in the body and this process no longer takes place. Unless an adequate amount of protein is eaten as soon as the treatment is over, protein deficiency is bound to develop, and this inevitably causes the marked retention of water known as hunger- edema.

The treatment is very simple. The patient is told to eat two eggs for breakfast and a huge steak for lunch and dinner followed by a large helping of cheese and to phone through the weight the next morning. When these instructions are followed a stunned voice is heard to report that two lbs. have vanished overnight, that the ankles are normal but that sleep was disturbed, owing to an extraordinary need to pass large quantities of water. The patient having learned this lesson usually has no further trouble.

Relapses

As a general rule one can say that 60%-70% of our cases experience little or no difficulty in holding their weight permanently. Relapses may be due to negligence in the basic rule of daily weighing. Many patients think that this is unnecessary and that they can judge any increase from the fit of their clothes. Some do not carry their scale with them on a journey as it is cumbersome and takes a big bite out of their luggage-allowance when flying. This is a disastrous mistake, because after a course of HCG as much as 10 lbs. can be regained without any noticeable change in the fit of the clothes. The reason for this is that after treatment newly acquired fat is at first evenly distributed and does not show the former preference for certain parts of the body.

Pregnancy or the menopause may annul the effect of a previous treatment. Women who take treatment during the one year after the last menstruation - that is at the onset of the menopause - do just as well as others, but among them the relapse rate is higher until the menopause is fully established. The period of one year after the last menstruation applies only to women who are not being treated with ovarian hormones. If these are taken, the premenopausal period may be indefinitely prolonged.

Late teenage girls who suffer from attacks of compulsive eating have by far the worst record of all as far as relapses are concerned.

Patients who have once taken the treatment never seem to hesitate to come back for another short course as soon as they notice that their weight is once again getting out of hand. They come quite cheerfully and hopefully, assured that they can be helped again. Repeat courses are often even more satisfactory than the first treatment and have the advantage, as do second courses, which the patient already knows he will feel comfortable throughout.

Plan of a Normal Course

125 I.U. of HCG daily (except during menstruation) until 40 injections have been given. - Until 3rd injection forced feeding.

After 3rd injection, 500 Calorie diet to be continued until 72 hours after the last injection.

For the following 3 weeks, all foods allowed except starch and sugar in any form (careful with very sweet fruit).

After 3 weeks, very gradually add starch in small quantities, always controlled by morning weighing.

CONCLUSION

The HCG + diet method can bring relief to every case of obesity, but the method is not simple. It is very time consuming and requires perfect cooperation between physician and patient. Each case must be handled individually, and the physician must have time to answer questions, allay fears and remove misunderstandings. He must also check the patient daily. When something goes wrong he must at once investigate until he finds the reason for any gain that may have occurred. In most cases it is useless to hand the patient a diet-sheet and let the nurse give him a "shot."

The method involves a highly complex bodily mechanism, and even though our theory may be wrong the physician must make himself some sort of picture of what is actually happening; otherwise he will not be able to deal with such difficulties as may arise during treatment.

I must beg those trying the method for the first time to adhere very strictly to the technique and the interpretations here outlined and thus treat a few hundred cases before embarking on experiments of their own, and until then refrain from introducing innovations, however thrilling they may seem. In a new method, innovations or departures from the original technique can only be usefully evaluated against a substantial background of experience with what is at the moment the orthodox procedure.

I have tried to cover all the problems that come to my mind. Yet a bewildering array of new questions keeps arising, and my interpretations are still fluid. In particular, I have never had an opportunity of conducting the laboratory investigations which are so necessary for a theoretical understanding of clinical observations, and I can only hope that those more fortunately placed will in time be able to fill this gap.

The problems of obesity are perhaps not as dramatic as the problems of cancer, or polio, but they often cause life long suffering. How many promising careers have been ruined by excessive fat; how many lives have been shortened.

If some way -however cumbersome - can be found to cope effectively with this universal problem of modern civilized man, our world will be a happier place for countless fellow men and women.

GLOSSARY

ACNE . . . Common skin disease in which pimples, often containing pus, appear on face, neck and shoulders.

ACTH . . . Abbreviation for adrenocorticotrophic hormone. One of the many hormones produced by the anterior lobe of the pituitary gland. ACTH controls the outer part, rind or cortex of the adrenal glands. When ACTH is injected it dramatically relieves arthritic pain, but it has many undesirable side effects, among which is a condition similar to severe obesity. ACTH is now usually replaced by cortisone.

ADRENALIN . . . Hormone produced by the inner part of the Adrenals. Among many other functions, adrenalin is concerned with blood pressure, emotional stress, fear and cold.

ADRENALS . . . Endocrine glands. Small bodies situated atop the kidneys and hence also known as suprarenal glands. The adrenals have an outer rind or cortex which produces vitally important hormones, among which are Cortisone similar substances. The adrenal cortex is controlled by ACTH. The inner part of the adrenals, the medulla, secretes adrenalin and is chiefly controlled by the autonomous nervous system.

ADRENOCORTEX... See adrenals.

AMPHETAMINES . . . Synthetic drugs which reduce the awareness of hunger and stimulate mental activity, rendering sleep impossible. When used for the latter two purposes they are dangerously habit-forming. They do not diminish the body's need for food, but merely suppress the perception of that need. The original drug was known as Benzedrine, from which modern variants such as Dexedrine, Dexamil, and Preludin, etc., have been derived. Amphetamines may help an obese patient to prevent a further increase in weight but are unsatisfactory for reducing, as they do not cure the underlying disorder and as their prolonged use may lead to malnutrition and addiction.

ARTERIOSCLEROSIS . . . Hardening of the arterial wall through the calcification of abnormal deposits of a fatlike substance known as cholesterol.

ASCHHIEIM-ZONDEK . . . Authors of a test by which early pregnancy can be diagnosed by injecting a woman's urine into female mice. The HCG present in pregnancy urine produces certain changes in the vagina of these animals. Many similar tests, using other animals such as rabbits, frogs, etc. have been devised.

ASSIMILATE . . . Absorb digested food from the intestines.

AUTONOMOUS . . . Here used to describe the independent or vegetative nervous system which manages the automatic regulations of the body.

BASAL METABOLISM . . . The body's chemical turnover at complete rest and when fasting. The basal metabolic rate is expressed as the amount of oxygen used up in a given time. The basal metabolic rate (BMR) is controlled by the thyroid gland.

CALORIE . . . The physicist's calorie is the amount of heat required to raise the temperature of 1 cc. of water by 1 degree Centigrade. The dieticiari's Calorie (always written with a capital C) is 1000 times greater. Thus when we speak of a 500 Calorie diet this means that the body is being supplied with as much fuel as would be required to raise the temperature of 500 liters of water by 1 degree Centigrade or 50 liters by 10 degrees. This is quite insufficient to cover the heat and energy requirements of an adult body. In the HCG method the deficit is made up from the abnormal fat-deposits, of which 1 lb. furnishes the body with more than 2000 Calories. As this is roughly the amount lost every day, a patient under HCG is never short of fuel.

CEREBRAL . . . Of the brain. Cerebral vascular disease is a disorder concerning the blood vessels of the brain, such as cerebral thrombosis or hemorrhage, known as apoplexy or stroke.

CHOLESTEROL . . . A fatlike substance contained in almost every cell of the body. In the blood it exists in two forms, known as free and esterified. The latter form is under certain conditions deposited in the inner lining of the arteries (see arteriosclerosis). No clear and definite relationship between fat intake and cholesterol-level in the blood has yet been established.

CHORIONIC . . . Of the chorion, which is part of the placenta or after-birth. The term chorionic is justly applied to HCG, as this hormone is exclusively produced in the placenta, from where it enters the human mother's blood and is later excreted in her urine.

COMPULSIVE EATING. . . A form of oral gratification with which a repressed sex-instinct is sometimes vicariously relieved. Compulsive eating must not be confused with the real hunger from which most obese patients suffer.

CONGENITAL . . . Any condition which exists at or before birth.

CORONARY ARTERIES . . . Two blood vessels which encircle the heart and supply all the blood required by the heart-muscle.

CORPUS LUTEUM . . . A yellow body which forms in the ovary at the follicle from which an egg has been detached. This body acts as an endocrine gland and plays an important role in menstruation and pregnancy. Its secretion is one of the sex hormones, and it is stimulated by another hormone known as LSH, which stands for luteum stimulating hormones. LSH is produced in the anterior lobe of the pituitary gland. LSH is truly gonadotrophic and must never be confused with HCG, which is a totally different substance, having no direct action on the corpus luteum.

CORTEX . . . Outer covering or rind. The term is applied to the outer part of the adrenals but is also used to describe the gray matter which covers the white matter of the brain.

CORTISONE . . . A synthetic substance which acts like an adrenal hormone. It is today used in the treatment of a large number of illnesses, and several chemical variants have been produced, among which are prednisone and triamcinolone.

CUSHING . . . A great American brain surgeon who described a condition of extreme obesity associated with symptoms of adrenal disorder. Cushing's Syndrome may be caused by organic disease of the pituitary or the adrenal glands but, as was later discovered, it also occurs as a result of excessive ACTH medication.

DIENCEPHALON . . . A primitive and hence very old part of the brain which lies between and under the two large hemispheres. In man the diencephalon (or hypothalamus) is subordinate to the higher brain or cortex, and yet it ultimately controls all that happens inside the body. It regulates all the endocrine glands, the autonomous nervous system, the turnover of fat and sugar. It seems also to be the seat of the primitive animal instincts and is the relay station at which emotions are translated into bodily reactions.

DIURETIC. . . Any substance that increases the flow of urine.

DYSFUNCTION . . . Abnormal functioning of any organ, be this excessive, deficient or in any way altered.

EDEMA . . . An abnormal accumulation of water in the tissues.

ELECTROCARDIOGRAM . . . Tracing of electric phenomena taking place in the heart during each beat. The tracing provides information about the condition and working of the heart which is not otherwise obtainable.

ENDOCRINE . . . We distinguish endocrine and exocrine glands. The former produce hormones, chemical regulators, which they secrete directly into the blood circulation in the gland and from where they are carried all over the body. Examples of endocrine glands are the pituitary, the thyroid and the adrenals. Exocrine glands produce a visible secretion such as saliva, sweat, urine. There are also glands which are endocrine and exocrine. Examples are the testicles, the prostate and the pancreas, which produces the hormone insulin and digestive ferments which flow from the gland into the intestinal tract. Endocrine glands are closely inter dependent of each other, they are linked to the autonomous nervous system and the diencephalon presides over this whole incredibly complex regulatory system.

EMACIATED . . . Grossly undernourished.

EUPHORIA . . . A feeling of particular physical and mental well being.

FERAL . . . Wild, unrestrained.

FIBROID . . . Any benign new growth of connective tissue. When such a tumor originates from a muscle, it is known as a myoma. The most common seat of myomas is the uterus.

FOLLICLE . . . Any small bodily cyst or sac containing a liquid. Here the term applies to the ovarian cyst in which the egg is formed. The egg is expelled when a ripe follicle bursts and this is known as ovulation (see corpus luteurn).

FSH . . . Abbreviation for follicle-stimulating hormone. FSH is another (see corpus luteum) anterior pituitary hormone which acts directly on the ovarian follicle and is therefore correctly called a gonadotrophin.

GLANDS . . . See endocrine.

GONADOTROPHIN . . . See corpus luteum, follicle and FSH. Gonadotrophic literally means sex gland-directed. FSH, LSH and the equivalent hormones in the male, all produced in the anterior lobe of the pituitary gland, are true gonadotrophins. Unfortunately and confusingly, the term gonadotrophin has also been applied to the placental hormone of pregnancy known as human chorionic gonadotrophin (HCG). This hormone acts on the diencephalon and can only indirectly influence the sex-glands via the anterior lobe of the pituitary.

HCG . . . Abbreviation for human chorionic gonadotrophin

HORMONES . . . See endocrine.

HYPERTENSION . . . High blood pressure.

HYPOGLYCEMIA . . . A condition in which the blood sugar is below normal. It can be relieved by eating sugar.

HYPOPHYSIS . . . Another name for the pituitary gland.

HYPOTHESIS . . . A tentative explanation or speculation on how observed facts and isolated scientific data can be brought into an intellectually satisfying relationship of cause and effect. Hypotheses are useful for directing further research, but they are not necessarily an exposition of what is believed to be the truth. Before a hypothesis can advance to the dignity of a theory or a law, it must be confirmed by all future research. As soon as research turns up data which no longer fit the hypothesis, it is immediately abandoned for a better one.

LSH . . . See corpus luteum.

METABOLISM . . . See basal metabolism.

MIGRAINE . . . Severe half-sided headache often associated with vomiting.

MUCOID . . . Slime-like.

MYOCARDIUM . . . The heart-muscle.

MYOMA . . . See fibroid.

MYXEDEMA . . . Accumulation of a mucoid substance in the tissues which occurs in cases of severe primary thyroid deficiency.

NEOLITHIC . . . In the history of human culture we distinguish the Early Stone Age or Paleolithic, the Middle Stone Age or Mesolithic and the New Stone Age or Neolithic period. The Neolithic period started about 8000 years ago when the first attempts at agriculture, pottery and animal domestication made at the end of the Mesolithic period suddenly began to develop rapidly along the road that led to modern civilization.

NORMAL SALINE . . . A low concentration of salt in water equal to the salinity of body fluids.

PHLEBITIS . . . An inflammation of the veins. When a blood-clot forms at the site of the inflammation, we speak of thrombophlebitis.

PITUITARY . . . A very complex endocrine gland which lies at the base of the skull, consisting chiefly of an anterior and a posterior lobe. The pituitary is controlled by the diencephalon, which regulates the anterior lobe by means of hormones which reach it through small blood vessels. The posterior lobe is controlled by nerves which run from the diencephalon into this part of the gland. The anterior lobe secretes many hormones, among which are those that regulate other glands such as the thyroid, the adrenals and the sex glands.

PLACENTA . . . The after-birth. In women, a large and highly complex organ through which the child in the womb receives its nourishment from the mother's body. It is the organ in which HCG is manufactured and then given off into the mother's blood.

PROTEIN . . . The living substance in plant and animal cells. Herbivorous animals can thrive on plant protein alone, but man must have some protein of animal origin (milk, eggs or flesh) to live healthily. When insufficient protein is eaten, the body retains water.

PSORIASIS . . . A skin disease which produces scaly patches. These tend to disappear during pregnancy and during the treatment of obesity by the HCG method.

RENAL . . . Of the kidney.

RESERPINE . . . An Indian drug extensively used in the treatment of high blood pressure and some forms of mental disorder.

RETENTION ENEMA . . . The slow infusion of a liquid into the rectum, from where it is absorbed and not evacuated.

SACRUM . . . A fusion of the lower vertebrate into the large bony mass to which the pelvis is attached.

SEDIMENTATION RATE . . . The speed at which a suspension of red blood cells settles out. A rapid settling out is called a high sedimentation rate and may be indicative of a large number of bodily disorders of pregnancy.

SEXUAL SELECTION . . . A sexual preference for individuals which show certain traits. If this preference or selection goes on generation after generation, more and more individuals showing the trait will appear among the general population. The natural environment has little or nothing to do with this process. Sexual selection therefore differs from natural selection, to which modern man is no longer subject because he changes his environment rather than let the environment change him.

STRIATION . . . Tearing of the lower layers of the skin owing to rapid stretching in obesity or during pregnancy. When first formed striae are dark reddish lines which later change into white scars.

SUPRARENAL GLANDS . . . See adrenals.

SYNDROME . . . A group of symptoms which in their association are characteristic of a particular disorder.

THROMBOPHLEBITIS . . . See phlebitis.

THROMBUS . . . A blood-clot in a blood-vessel.

TRIAMCINOLONE . . . A modern derivative of cortisone.

URIC ACID . . . A product of incomplete protein-breakdown or utilization in the body. When uric acid becomes deposited in the gristle of the joints we speak of gout.

VARICOSE ULCERS . . . Chronic ulceration above the ankles due to varicose veins which interfere with the normal blood circulation in the affected areas.

VEGETATIVE . . . See autonomous.

VERTEBRATE . . . Any animal that has a back-bone.